ABOVE THE CUT

ABOVE THE CUT

LEGENDS OF MODERN SURGERY

hachette
INDIA

First published as *Legends of Modern Surgery* in 2021
by Hachette India
(Registered name: Hachette Book Publishing India Pvt. Ltd)
An Hachette UK company
www.hachetteindia.com

1

This trade edition first published in 2022

Compiled and edited by Hansa Makhijani Jain

This book was also supplied as a limited (not for sale) custom gift edition with the title *Legends of Surgery*

ISBN 978-93-5009-598-0

Hachette Book Publishing India Pvt. Ltd
4th & 5th Floors, Corporate Centre,
Plot No. 94, Sector 44, Gurugram 122003, India

Typeset in Sabon LT Std 11.5/16.5
by R. Ajith Kumar, New Delhi

Printed and bound in India by Manipal Technologies Limited, Manipal

FSC www.fsc.org MIX Paper from responsible sources FSC™ C043100

‘The physician should look upon the patient as a besieged city and try to rescue him with every means that art and science place at his command.’

– ALEXANDER OF TRALLES

CONTENTS

ONE

20 PIONEERS OF MODERN SURGERY

PEEPING INSIDE THE STATE-OF-THE-ART OPERATING theatres of today, it is hard to imagine a time when surgery was primitive. In medieval Europe, the tough work of surgery was the domain of barbers. It took a while for surgery to leave their hands and become a separate professionalized realm. In 1689, the barber-surgeons guild received the exclusive right to examine barber-surgeons and, in 1755, the control of all surgeons in the country. According to a paper published in a Swedish medical journal entitled 'From Barber to Surgeon – The Process of Professionalization', 'The guild developed their own set of ethics and office oaths. The quality of the training increased to a higher level with the establishment of professorships outside the universities with the task to train barber-surgeons was made. The craft organization, which from the end of the 17th century was called the Society of Surgeons, received several instructions from the King.' These surgeons primarily served the army and navy, addressing surgical requirements and tending to big and small wounds. They had no professional or academic training. Any semblance of organized training would only be realized in the 19th century after the dissolution of the Society of Surgeons in 1797. The Age of Enlightenment (1715–89) also saw tremendous progress in surgical procedures.

To make matters more complicated, there was also no recorded use of ether anaesthesia till 1846 and the patient had to be pinned down by strong, muscular attendants whose job was to completely disregard the patient's cries and screams and keep them as still as possible for the convenience of the doctor. Whether the surgery was major or minor, the patient would be wide awake for the procedure. Chloroform and nitrous oxide (laughing gas) were used before the acceptance of ether anaesthesia.

It was also a time before hygiene practices such as sterilized operation theatres became mainstays. The thorough washing of hands and surgical tools was considered optional. Doctors would strut about with pride in bloodstained gowns after a surgical procedure to signify their prowess and experience. Lab coats and bed linen would only be washed before being put away for storage. On all patients, the same probe would be used during hospital rounds to look for undrained pus in their wounds. More patients lost their lives due to post-surgery infections rather than the surgical procedure itself. Septic complications were such a grave cause of concern that there was even talk of banning all surgical procedures, especially those on the chest, abdomen and brain. That was then. Today, even the most complicated surgeries have been finely tuned to safe, effective and reliable techniques. Surgeons from different streams of medicine have contributed immensely to make surgery what it is today.

[1]

JOSEPH LISTER

A pioneer of antiseptic surgery, Dr Joseph Lister's insightful forays into bacteriology and infection in wounds earned him the title of the father of modern surgery. Though his surgical techniques were average at best, his research paved the way for modern, sterile surgery throughout the world. Post-operative infections could be minimized with his techniques, making surgeries much safer for patients and easier to manage for surgeons. No wonder he has been regarded as 'the greatest surgical benefactor to mankind' in *The Cambridge Illustrated History of Surgery*.

Lister was born into a Quaker family in Essex, England, and was the second of six siblings. Many believe that he inherited the spirit of innovation from his father Joseph Jackson Lister, who was elected a Fellow of the Royal Society for coming up with the first achromatic lens. He also co-authored a paper with Thomas Hodgkin about red blood cells. His mother, Isabella Lister, also had an academic bend of mind as she used to work in a school, where her widowed mother was a superintendent, before she got married. However, it was his father who had a major influence on him while growing up. His father's microscope would act as one of the early apparatuses he used for examining dissections on small animals – a result of his eager interest in natural history. Throughout various junctures in Lister's career, he would often seek his father's opinion.

He completed his medical education at the University College of the University of London and became house surgeon at the University College Hospital. Here, he would earn a fellowship from the Royal College of Surgeons. He studied under and assisted the renowned surgeon James Syme in Edinburgh, where he made the acquaintance of his daughter Agnes Syme, who also had a keen interest in science. The two would go on to marry and Agnes would become Lister's lab partner for all their years to come.

During his time teaching surgery at the University of Glasgow in Scotland, Lister came to know about a much-talked about paper by the French chemist Louis Pasteur. He had illustrated that food spoilage could occur under anaerobic conditions if microorganisms were present, and recommended three methods to eradicate the microorganisms: filtration, exposure to heat or exposure to chemical solutions. This intrigued Lister and he began experimenting with the aim of using the same principles to develop antiseptic techniques for treating wounds. Since the first two of Pasteur's approaches were not feasible for the treatment of human tissue, Lister experimented with the third. He took inspiration from another chemist's work for this: Friedlieb Ferdinand Runge, a German chemist, had discovered phenol or carbolic acid in 1834. Lister was curious about the efficacy of carbolic acid when applied directly to wounds. He also started spraying surgical instruments and dressings with a carbolic acid solution. He was astonished to see a remarkable reduction in the occurrence of gangrene when the solution was directly dabbed on wounds. Lister began writing about his findings in medical journals. In 1867, a series of six articles were published in *The Lancet*. He also insisted on surgeons working under him to wear clean gloves and wash their hands with a 5 per cent carbolic acid solution.

According to a 2012 article published in the *Canadian Journal of Surgery*, at the Dublin meeting of the British Medical Association in August 1867, Lister stated 'previous to its introduction, the 2 large wards in which most of my cases of accident and of operation are treated were amongst the unhealthiest in the whole of surgical division at the Glasgow Royal Infirmary... but since the antiseptic treatment has been brought into full operation... my wards... have completely changed their character; so that during the last 9 months not a single instance of pyaemia, hospital gangrene or erysipelas has occurred in them.'

Though Lister's research and experiments ushered in a new era in surgery, at the time of his discoveries, his ideas were not well received. His ideas would be subjected to ridicule and mockery at conferences while *The Lancet*, which had initially published his findings, warned the medical fraternity in 1873 against his groundbreaking work. Germany was the first nation to embrace Lister's germ theory, followed by the United States and France. His own country joined in the enthusiasm only later, once the results of his work were clearly noticeable among patients. Awards and accolades followed. For several years, he served Queen Victoria as a Surgeon Extraordinary and the royal household as a senior surgeon. A memorial to him sits in Portland Place in London, while Glasgow honoured him with a statue at Kelvingrove Park.

At the age of 84 in February 1912, Lister died an accomplished man, having changed the future of surgery.

[2]
DANIEL HALE WILLIAMS

Not only was Dr Daniel Hale Williams the first successful heart surgeon in recorded history, he was also a pioneer in racial equality in the medical fraternity. The son of a Scots-Irish and Black barber father and an African American mother, Williams was the first to set up the first Black-owned interracial hospital in America. Born in 1856 in Hollidaysburg, Pennsylvania, Williams was just nine years old when his father succumbed to tuberculosis. With seven children to manage, his mother found it a challenge to make ends meet, often moving cities and sending some of the children to live with relatives. Williams apprenticed with a shoemaker and later also opened a barber shop with his sister in Edgerton, Wisconsin. But his heart was neither in shoes nor in the barber shop. He knew he wanted more: an education.

However, with their limited means, getting an extensive education was a challenge. At the age of 20, Williams started working as an apprentice under Dr Henry W. Palmer. After two years, he was able to support himself through medical college at Northwestern University Medical School, which was known as Chicago Medical College at the time. After graduating in 1883, he set up his own private practice in Chicago while also serving as a surgeon for the South Side Dispensary and a physician for the Protestant Orphan Asylum. He also taught anatomy at his alma mater and served as surgeon to the City Railway Company. In 1889, he was appointed to the state's board of health by the governor of Illinois. He decided to venture into private practice as black doctors were not allowed to work in private hospitals at the time. His medical office was open to both white and black patients and he was sincerely motivated to bridge the gap between the races. His dream was realized in 1891, when he founded Provident Hospital in Chicago with the aim of providing accessible and quality healthcare to African Americans in the city. Like his clinic, however, the hospital was also open to all races and had an integrated staff. Now a public hospital, it also offered a training residency for doctors and training school for nurses.

The turning point in the surgeon's career came in 1893, when James Cornish was admitted to Provident Hospital at night. He had been stabbed directly through the left fifth costal cartilage and began to show symptoms of shock in the morning. After inspecting the wound between two ribs, Williams cut the rib cartilage, creating a small trapdoor to the heart. The left internal mammary artery had been damaged and was duly sutured. The pericardium (sac around the heart) also had a gash from the knife near the right coronary artery. With the heart beating and no possibility of a transfusion, the surgeon rinsed the wound with salt solution. As his assistants observed, Williams took hold of the edges of the palpitating wound with his forceps, and stitched them together. He conducted a separate procedure to drain fluid. After about 50 days since his arrival, Cornish walked out of the hospital, his heartbeat normal. He lived for another 20 years.

According to *Encyclopaedia Britannica*, 'although contemporary medical opinion disapproved of surgical treatment of heart wounds, Williams opened the patient's thoracic cavity without aid of blood transfusions or modern anesthetics and antibiotics... Williams's procedure is cited as the first recorded repair of the pericardium; some sources, however, cite a similar operation performed by H.C. Dalton of St. Louis in 1891.'

Williams received honorary degrees from Howard and Wilberforce Universities and was also the only African

American to be elected a charter member of the American College of Surgeons. He died in 1931, at the age of 75, after suffering a stroke.

[3]
HARVEY CUSHING

A pioneer of brain surgery, Harvey Cushing is known for his exhaustive and meticulous documentation of the clinical and pathological features of cerebral tumours and for pioneering the basic methods and techniques of operative surgery on the brain, which are now standard practice. He was also the first medical professional to define Cushing's disease, an endocrine disorder that was subsequently named after him. The survival rate of patients after difficult operations for intracranial tumours became higher with his techniques. Cushing was the first to use X-rays to diagnose brain tumours. He employed electrical stimuli to explore the human sensory cortex and played a crucial role in the development of the Bovie electrocautery tool with physicist William T. Bovie. His achievements also include the introduction of the concept of blood pressure management to North America. According to a 2017 issue of *Journal of the Intensive Care Society*, 'His extraordinary medical career spanning over 40 years, including operating on over 2,000 brain tumours, and his discoveries and innovations, have helped make neurology and neurosurgery the respected specialties they are now.'

Born in 1869 in Cleveland, Ohio, to Elizabeth Maria Williams and physician Henry Kirke Cushing, he was the youngest of ten siblings. His interest in science and medicine was nurtured by the Cleveland Manual Training School, where unique programmes, such as the training in manual dexterity, would prove to be handy in honing Cushing's surgical skills later. After graduating with a Bachelor of Arts degree in 1891 from Yale University, he went on to study medicine at Harvard Medical School and earned his medical degree in 1895. An internship at Massachusetts General Hospital followed. Cushing got a brilliant opportunity when he secured a residency in surgery under the able guidance of legendary surgeon William Stewart Halsted at the Johns Hopkins Hospital in Baltimore, Maryland.

In 1900, Cushing found himself in Europe, working with greats such as Sir Victor Horsley. He had the great fortune of working closely with Nobel Prize winners Emil Theodor Kocher in Bern, Switzerland and Sir Charles Scott Sherrington in Liverpool, England. According to a feature in a 2016 issue of *Neurology India*, 'His association with Kocher was the turning point in his career, and it was in his laboratory that he met Victor Krönecker, the physiologist, and started working on the effects of raised intracranial tension on respiratory rate, pulse rate, and blood pressure which was to earn him world-wide renown. The reflex earned the eponymous name, the *Cushing's response*. With Sherrington, he worked on the effects of electrical excitability of the cerebral cortex in primates.'

After gaining all that insight and experience in Europe, Cushing returned to Baltimore and started his own private practice. He soon had his hands full as he was appointed as an associate professor of surgery at Johns Hopkins Hospital. He was only 32 and was in complete charge of all surgeries involving the central nervous system. He became surgeon-in-chief at the Peter Bent Brigham Hospital in Boston in 1911 and a professor of surgery at the Harvard Medical School the next year. Cushing emerged as one of the world's leading teachers of neurosurgery during his time and immensely helped organize and shape the specialty. He acquired an international reputation in America and Europe and was made an honorary fellow of the Royal College of Surgeons, London, in 1913. He was also elected a fellow of the American Academy of Arts and Sciences in 1914. Among other awards and accolades, Cushing received the Cameron Prize for Therapeutics of the University of Edinburgh in 1924. For a couple of years during the First World War, Cushing served first as a Major, then as Lieutenant Colonel, and subsequently Colonel. He returned to civilian practice in 1919 and, in 1923, was awarded the Distinguished Service Medal by the United States Army.

Cushing was passionate about documenting his profession and wrote extensively on surgery of the brain and spinal column. Later in his career, he wrote the Pulitzer Prize-winning biography of Canadian physician Sir William Osler, which was published in 1925. Until his retirement in 1937, he taught neurology at Yale School of Medicine, earning the highest academic rank of Sterling Professor.

Cushing died in 1939, in his 71st year, of a myocardial infarction. He was survived by his wife Katharine Stone Crowell and their five children.

[4]
DWIGHT EMARY HARKEN

The Intensive Care Unit (ICU) that saves multiple lives, aiding the recovery of vulnerable patients every day around the globe, was the brainchild of Dwight Emary Harken. The American surgical giant was a pioneering heart surgeon. He is also known for developing the first device to help the heart pump. His work with the implantation of artificial aortic and mitral valves is also revered. In fact, Harken is regarded by many as the father of cardiac surgery.

Born in the small town of Osceola, Iowa, in 1910, Harken was drawn to the medical profession from an early age. He had a physician father to look up to. After receiving his bachelor's and medical degrees from

Harvard, he was off to New York's Bellevue Hospital. He went on to do postgraduate studies at the Royal Brompton Hospital in London, working with the famous thoracic surgeon Arthur Tudor Edwards.

The 'eureka moment' of Harken's career, however, came on the war front when he was serving as a Lieutenant Colonel in the US Army Medical Corps. During the Normandy invasion in 1944, he found an interesting way to remove shrapnel from the heart. He would cut into the wall of a beating heart and then use his finger to locate and remove the shrapnel. He operated on 134 soldiers without losing a single one. According to a 2018 article in the journal of the Baylor University Medical Center, 'Techniques at that time were primitive and, of course, there was no heart-lung machine. He would therefore make a hole in the heart or blood vessel, remove the foreign body, and then suture it rapidly with the blood spurting up to the ceiling! The operation required nerves of steel and stamina, qualities that Dwight must have had after being an amateur boxer.' Such bravado obviously garnered a great deal of attention and appreciation from the medical fraternity. Dr Richard Meade called it the greatest technical advance in chest surgery during World War II, while Dr Frank B. Berry called this series 'the first consistently successful operations in this area'.

After the war, he joined Harvard professor Elliott Cutler's staff. Cutler had managed to successfully open stenoses of the mitral valve in 1923 with an instrument invented by him. Harken introduced a cardiovalvulotome, given to him by Cutler, through the left auricle and into the heart of a 27-year-old patient with grave mitral stenosis in 1948. Only six days earlier, Charles Bailey in Philadelphia had achieved a similar feat. However, with Harken publishing his results first, a battle over who did it first ensued. Bailey named his technique valvotomy, while Dwight referred to it as valvuloplasty. Both methods of operation were similar; however, Dwight almost gave up hope after losing six patients in a row. But with some help from Cutler, he was given a final chance. His seventh patient turned things around and there was no looking back. According to the journal of the Baylor University Medical Center, after 500 operations the mortality rate was a negligible 0.6 per cent.

In June 1960, he implanted the first stainless steel cage prosthesis, which was also developed by him. His first patient survived 20 years after the surgery. He was also one of the key figures involved in the implantation of the first pacemakers at the Peter Bent Brigham Hospital at Harvard. Arguably, his greatest achievement was coming up with the concept of intensive care. Realizing that the first few hours after surgery can make or break the situation when it comes to recovery of the patient, he began organizing such units. The idea was a success and ICUs, as we now call them, mushroomed everywhere across the globe.

Harken had an extensive career as an academic and

taught for many years at Harvard, nurturing several surgeons par excellence. He died in 1993 and was described as 'the father of heart surgery' by the *New York Times* in his obituary.

[5]
HERMANN SCHLOFFER

One wouldn't expect an abdominal surgeon to perform a surgery on a pituitary adenoma. But that's what Hermann Schloffer did in 1907. At the University of Innsbruck, the Austrian surgeon performed the first transsphenoidal surgery on a patient suffering from a pituitary adenoma, using a superior nasal route via a transfacial lateral rhinotomy incision. Notwithstanding the technological limitations of his time, Schloffer's surgery was path-breaking and paved the way for future development and fine-tuning of transsphenoidal pituitary surgery. The surgery, which was his greatest contribution to neurosurgery, in turn, influenced eminent surgeons such as Oskar Hirsch, Theodor Kocher and Harvey Cushing. The transsphenoidal approach has gone through a number of modifications and still remains the favoured approach for lesions of the sella turcica till today.

This first patient, a 30-year-old man with a 6-year history of decreasing vision and worsening headaches, survived the surgery and showed remarkable improvement.

His visual field defects, appetite, sleep pattern and subjective muscle strength, all appeared to become better. Unfortunately, a little over two months after the surgery, the patient died after a seizure, throbbing headaches, vomiting, bradycardia and hypothermia. According to a 2012 feature in the journal *Neurosurgical Focus*, 'An autopsy revealed extensive residual tumor compressing the foramen of Monro, with enlarged lateral ventricles. A diagnosis of hydrocephalus was given as the cause of the patient's death, ultimately the result of incomplete tumor resection.' There were lessons to be learned and Schloffer acknowledged this, stating, 'In the future it will be more correct to not attach too much significance to the larger tumors resting on the saddle and X-rays of these larger tumors because much of the tumor may have grown out considerably from the sella and sellar entrance.'

While the patient eventually died, the surgery was considered a success because it was able to provide symptomatic relief from the sufferings. Schloffer ascribed the unsatisfactory outcome to technological limitations and his own reluctance to probe the sella aggressively or excise the pituitary excessively. 'Radiological imaging was still in its infancy, and one of its major shortcomings included its difficulty in accurately establishing the exact size and position of intracranial soft tissue masses, a problem that was not resolved until 12 years later with the development of pneumoencephalography in 1919,' according to the *Neurosurgical Focus* feature.

Born in 1869 in Graz in Styria, Austria, Schloffer completed his medical education at the University of Freiburg and University of Graz, earning his medical doctorate in 1892. He was employed as a surgical assistant and associate professor in Prague. In 1903, he worked as a surgeon and professor at the University of Innsbruck. Here, he played a crucial role in establishing a department of oral surgery under the direction of the board of the dental institute. In 1911, he returned to the Charles University of Prague as a professor of surgery, where he had had a brief stint in the early years of his career.

Schloffer was also the first to remove a spleen for Idiopathic Thrombocytopenic Purpura (ITP) in 1916. The surgery was based on his student Paul Kaznelson's idea that to put a stop to the extreme destruction of platelets in ITP that occurs in the spleen, a splenectomy should be performed. Schloffer followed his student's suggestion and the first patient to undergo this treatment for chronic ITP showed promising results.

He also coined the terms 'Schloffer tumour' and 'Schloffer broth' for a rare pseudotumour stemming from chronic granulomatous inflammation secondary to scarring from abdominal surgeries and a urine agar used for the cultivation of Corynebacterium diptheriae, respectively.

Much like his lawyer father, Schloffer was an active member of Austrian high society and was part of several prestigious organizations such as the Society for the Support of German Arts, Research, and Literature, Society of Physicians in Vienna, Correspondents of Medical Societies in Innsbruck and Budapest. The greatest honour bestowed on him was the third class medal of the Order of Emperor Franz Josef I.

He died in 1937 at the age of 68.

[6]
SIR HAROLD GILLIES

Necessity is the mother of invention, they say. Same was the case with Sir Harold Gillies, who after serving in the First World War and seeing so many lives ruined by facial disfigurement, decided to do something about it. Though he was a trained otolaryngologist, his contribution to reconstructive surgery earned him the title of the father of modern plastic surgery. Gillies was moved by the struggle of strong and brave men, whose confidence was crushed after sustaining severe facial deformities on the battlefront. While many soldiers would wear their battle scars as badges of honour, for those who had gone through facial disfigurement, it was a different matter altogether. Many with disfigured jaws and burnt skin would look so ghastly that it would be difficult for them to get jobs elsewhere, even as their injuries, and sometimes permanent disabilities, deemed them unfit for a future in the defence services.

That is not the price one should have to pay for serving one's country, Gillies felt. The fact that several of the techniques devised by him during the First World War are still used in modern reconstructive surgeries is a testament to his genius.

Born in 1882 in Dunedin, New Zealand, Gillies attended the Whanganui Collegiate School. He left his country to study medicine in England at the Gonville and Caius College, Cambridge, where he also proved to be a valuable sportsman, participating in golf and rowing. He would not return to New Zealand for over five decades and made England his home.

When the First World War began in 1914, Gillies joined the Royal Army Medical Corps, and in France, observed the horrific facial injuries and disfigurations sustained by soldiers. Seeing the work that dentist and oral surgeon Charles Valadier and the French surgeon Hippolyte Morestin were doing on the faces of the soldiers, he requested the War Office for a similar set-up on his return. With some assistance from Sir William Arbuthnot Lane, a pioneering cleft palate surgeon, he was allocated beds for such patients at the Cambridge Hospital, Aldershot. Gillies was also given permission to design and build a hutted hospital on the grounds of Frognal House, Sidcup, in order to address the casualties coming in from the Battle of Somme. It eventually became the Queen Mary's Hospital. According to a bulletin by the Royal College of Surgeons of England honouring

Gillies, the problems were enormous and encompassed horrendous facial wounds with major loss of soft tissue and bone, infection, and difficult anaesthesia – for it was not until nearly the end of the war that single-tube endotracheal anaesthesia was introduced by Gillies's one-time colleague, the Irish anaesthetist Sir Ivan Magill.

The article also stated, 'Gillies himself had been gleaning ideas on reconstruction from many sources, which he then put into practice to develop some overriding "principles" of management, as every wound was different. In most cases, in order to reduce the chance of infection the wounds were encouraged to heal before reconstruction. Skin grafts had limited use; mostly local or distant flaps were used. At the end of 1917 Gillies struck on the idea of the tube pedicle for transferring a bulk of tissue.' His observations and experiences were published in his book in 1920, *Plastic Surgery of the Face*. After the war, the set-up at Sidcup was no longer required. It was dismantled in 1925 and it was then all up to Gillies, along with his colleague Thomas Pomfret Kilner, to practice the new specialty of plastic surgery. For his work during the war, Gillies was knighted in 1930.

Visiting many hospitals in several states, Gillies tirelessly promoted and helped develop the specialty. Doctors would throng from many countries to study under him. He always stayed updated with the latest developments in surgery, developing many techniques for reconstructive surgery. He was a founder member of the British Association of Plastic Surgeons, becoming its first president in 1946.

His resourcefulness and vast experience with the specialty also proved to be of immense value in the first case of sex reassignment surgery in the country. His second book, co-written with facial reconstructive surgeon Ralph Millard, *The Principles and Art of Plastic Surgery*, was published in 1957 and proved to be a must-have for those in the profession. After a life of travelling, teaching and devoting his entire life to the development of plastic surgery, he passed away in 1960 at the age of 78, while he was still working.

[7]
JOHN HUNTER

If it weren't for John Hunter's rare passion for research, surgery would have been stuck in the dark for a much longer time. Interestingly, Hunter never studied medicine at any university and neither did he try to earn the title of a doctor, a common phenomenon for surgeons in the 18th century. In 1748, he simply went to London to assist his brother William in preparing dissections. William, a physician and obstetrician, taught a course of anatomy in London at the time. In the summers of 1749 and 1750, Hunter learned surgery from William Cheselden at Chelsea Hospital, while his winters were devoted to dissections with his brother. He also trained under Percivall Pott, picking up on the nuances of surgery.

Since he did not have any sort of formal training in any one specialty, he applied scientific conclusions to various concepts such as wound healing, transplantation, heart disease, orthopaedics and pathology. The specimens and notes he compiled later transformed into one of his greatest contributions to medicine: the Hunterian Museum.

Born in 1728 in Long Calderwood in Scotland, Hunter was the last of ten children. Exhibiting a strong distaste for the structured learning enforced at school, Hunter preferred to spend most of his childhood exploring the natural wonders of his father's estate in East Kilbride, Scotland. His fondness for the natural world would not leave him till his dying breath. Surprisingly, for someone who detested academics, Hunter proved to be quite adept at dissections in his brother's lab in London. After training at Chelsea Hospital in 1749 and an apprenticeship in surgery at St. Bartholomew's Hospital, Hunter would go on to work at St. George's Hospital. However, his stint didn't last long as he was consumed with his passion for anatomy and wanted to devote his entire time to it. He also served as an army surgeon in 1760, spending three years in France and Portugal. He worked on new ideas on the treatment strategies of common ailments like gunshot wounds and venereal disease, apart from continuing his exploration of the natural world and collecting specimens of several animals.

In 1763, after returning from the armed services, he invested in some land in Earl's Court in London, where he gathered animals of sundry species to expand his knowledge of comparative anatomy. He would eventually make this place his home with his wife – a poet – and their four children. He was one of the first in the medical profession to focus on the pathology of infectious conditions like tuberculosis, suppuration in abscesses, bone lesions and osteomyelitis. His years of hard work paid off when, in 1767, he was elected a fellow of the Royal Society. In 1768, he returned to St. George's Hospital as he was elected Surgeon. He moved to an enormous house in Leicester Square in 1783, which allowed him to take resident pupils. The ample space also gave him an opportunity to arrange his vast collection of specimens into a teaching museum. Almost 14,000 specimens of more than 500 different species of plants and animals were available to be observed at his museum.

By the 1780s, he had gained a reputation as a scientific surgeon and emerged as one of the top teachers of surgery. Hunter did not just restrict himself to human anatomy in lectures. Instead, he urged his students to explore the relationship between structure and function in all kinds of living beings. He insisted that surgeons will be able to treat their patients better if they comprehend how the body adapts to and compensates for damage due to injury, disease or environmental changes.

His stubborn and relentlessness pursuit of science earned him various prestigious accolades and honours that continued even after his demise. In 1776, King George III gave him the title of Surgeon Extraordinary. Hunter also received the revered Copley Medal from the Royal Society in 1786. He died in 1793 while engaged in an argument with the board of St. George's Hospital about training two students who had not been approved for the surgical profession. The Hunterian Museum at the Royal College of Surgeons houses his collection of anatomical specimens, while the Hunterian Society of London has been named in his honour. A bust of him had been placed near his home in Leicester Square, London, until its redesigning in 2010–12. A plaster cast medallion of John Hunter sits in London's Science Museum. His home country has also honoured him by preserving his birthplace in Long Calderwood, Scotland, as Hunter House Museum, while his statue can be viewed at the Scottish National Portrait Gallery.

[8]
WILLIAM EDWARDS LADD

Born in 1880 in Milton, Massachusetts, William Edwards Ladd was the sixth of seven children born to William Jones Ladd and his wife, Anna Russell Watson. Following in the footsteps of his father, he graduated with a BA from Harvard University in 1902, followed by an MD from Harvard Medical School in 1906. He served as an assistant visiting surgeon to the Boston City Hospital, Infant's Hospital, Children's Hospital and Milton Hospital from 1910 to 1913. He also became assistant professor in surgery at Harvard Medical School in 1912; later, he rose to the position of full professor. Though most of his training and practice revolved around adult surgery, things changed in 1917 after the Halifax ship explosion in Nova Scotia, Canada, on 6 December 1917. Ladd reached the site within 24 hours with a team of physicians and nurses to treat casualties, of whom hundreds were children who had suffered burns and lacerations.

Upon his return from Halifax, Ladd made a life-changing decision. He would no longer follow surgical practice in adult medicine. Instead, he would fully devote his time to the development of paediatric surgery. This would prove to be a difficult decision, as he had to deal with opposition from both paediatricians and surgeons, as they did not feel the need for a separate department for the management of children's diseases. According to a 2003 issue of the journal *Current Surgery*, he championed the now accepted view that children are not 'little adults', and trained a cadre of surgeons dedicated to their care. In 1927, he became surgeon-in-chief at the Boston Children's Hospital, where he would go on to set up a paediatric surgical training programme.

A 2013 article in the journal *the American Surgeon* comments on an article Ladd published in February 1932, entitled 'Congenital Obstruction of the Duodenum in Children': 'Although such cases had been described previously, this condition was often overlooked by doctors. In his article, Ladd described the embryological cause of the disease, attributing it to the incomplete rotation of the intestines, leading to the attachment of the cecum to the posterior abdominal wall by the "mesenteric attachments," resulting in duodenal obstruction. These attachments were later referred to as "Ladd bands". Because timely and appropriate surgical intervention offers the only chance for cure in these patients, Ladd emphasized that early suspicion for the disease is crucial.' The recovery rates of patients skyrocketed after the introduction of this technique.

Ladd wrote a textbook and several extensively researched papers on findings and new surgical techniques in paediatric surgery. He also pioneered the repair of cleft palates, bladder exstrophy and the surgical management of Wilms' tumour. He also made important contributions to the surgical repair of tracheoesophageal fistulas, biliary atresia, anorectal abnormalities, and oesophageal atresia. His name bears several medical eponyms such as the Ladd band and Ladd's syndrome among others. In addition, he groomed a generation of paediatric surgeons like Orvar Swenson and Robert E. Gross. Gross succeeded Ladd as Surgeon-in-Chief at Boston Children's Hospital on his retirement in 1945.

Ladd was a founding member of the American Academy of Pediatrics, American Board of Surgery, and the American Association of Plastic Surgeons. Memberships of prestigious groups such as the New England Surgical Society, the American College of Surgeons, and the American Surgical Association were also bestowed on him.

He spent his life treating children with great passion and devotion. He also extensively researched several children's diseases as individual entities, independent of their adult counterparts. Ladd passed away at the age of 86 in 1967, having changed the lives of countless children and their families.

[9]
BENJAMIN BELL

Benjamin Bell has gone down in history as the first of the famous Edinburgh scientific surgeons and for his 'save skin' approach to surgery that led to improved rates of wound healing in procedures like amputations and mastectomies. But perhaps he is best-known for his surgical textbook, *A System of Surgery*, which was considered the Bible for aspiring surgeons and continues to be in print today.

Born into an agricultural family in 1749 in Dumfries, Scotland, Bell was the eldest surviving child among 15 children. By the time he completed his schooling at the Dumfries Grammar School, he was sure he wanted a career in medicine. After schooling, he assisted surgeon James Hill in his hometown. In 1766, he was off to Edinburgh to study medicine at the Edinburgh University, where he enjoyed the good fortune of being taught by legendary teachers such as anatomist Alexander Monro and chemist Joseph Black. After a couple of years at the Edinburgh Royal Infirmary, he was elected a freeman surgeon-apothecary of the Incorporation of Surgeons of Edinburgh, which would later become the Royal College of Surgeons of Edinburgh. Making good use of his family's agricultural money, he set out for London and Paris to expand his horizons. It was a most exciting time in young Bell's life as he made the acquaintance of eminent surgeons and scientists such as Percivall Pott, Joseph Priestley, and John Hunter.

After gaining ample exposure, Bell returned to Edinburgh to practice surgery. At the age of 24, he was elected as one of four attendant surgeons at the Royal Infirmary of Edinburgh. He would hold this post for eighteen years, which was a feat, considering it was a rotation position. Many believe it was because of his friendship with James Gregory, an influential member on the Infirmary Board of Management. Bell met with an accident in 1775 when he fell from horseback. The accident rendered him unable to continue practicing his duties as a surgeon for around two years. However, he used his time resourcefully to write and indulge in farming. *The Theory and Management of Ulcers* was first published in 1778 and was well-received, eventually becoming a classic. Between 1783 and 1788, he released six volumes of *A System of Surgery*. It was an exhaustive work and became a bestseller, with several editions published in America, France, Italy, Spain, and Germany. In his 1793 treatise on venereal disease, he made the point that syphilis and gonorrhoea were not the same disease. He was not proven right for decades and his hypothesis was rubbished by mainstream medicine at the time.

After his forced sabbatical to recover from horseback injuries, Bell returned to practice, all set for the most successful period of his life. He collaborated with other Scottish surgeons such as James Gibson, James Russell, and Andrew Wardrop. In 1783, Bell became one of the founding fellows of the Royal Society of Edinburgh.

He passed away after an illustrious career in 1806 in Edinburgh.

[10]
THOMAS STARZL

One of the most cited scientists in the world, Thomas Starzl never intended to be a doctor or even study anything related to medicine. He wanted to be a priest. However, he was still destined to serve mankind, albeit in a different way. At the age of 21, Starzl's life plans changed when his mother passed away due to breast cancer in 1947. After stepping into his medical career, he would go on to introduce a liver transplantation programme, along with the use of a new drug that would make transplantation an accepted treatment for many ailments that were otherwise deemed hopeless. He performed the world's first liver transplant in 1963, followed by the world's first successful liver transplant in 1967, as well as the first simultaneous heart and liver transplantation in 1984.

Born in 1926, in Le Mars, Iowa, to newspaper editor and science fiction writer Roman Frederick Starzl and Anna Laura Fitzgerald, a teacher and nurse, Starzl completed his BSc in Biology from Westminster College in Fulton, Missouri. His next stop was the Northwestern University Medical School in Chicago, where he received a Master of Science degree in anatomy in 1950. Two years later, after spending an extra year at medical school, he earned both a PhD in neurophysiology and an MD with distinction. He worked first at Johns Hopkins Hospital in Baltimore and then at Jackson Memorial Hospital in Miami.

He moved to the University of Colorado in 1962 as a surgeon and researcher in organ transplantation, a field that was in its infancy at the time. According to *The BMJ*, the journal of the British Medical Association, he performed the first liver transplant in March 1963. 'His realisation that liver transplantation could be used in a variety of metabolic conditions had been triggered after conducting studies in dogs, exploring whether portal vein nutrients contribute to liver health. His first patient, a 3 year old boy with biliary atresia, bled to death during surgery.' His subsequent patients survived the surgery, but succumbed to multiple infections and pulmonary emboli within a few weeks. According to the 1965 issue of the journal *Surgery*, 'Surgeons worldwide declared a moratorium on the procedure, forcing Starzl back to the drawing board to devise new procedures, such as bypassing blood from the lower to the upper half of the recipient's body with plastic tubes; preventing ischaemic injury to donor livers by infusion with chilled solutions; control of blood coagulation; and immunosuppression.'

However, the surgeon did not lose heart. In 1967, he was finally successful with a patient – Julie Rodriguez, a one-year-old with liver cancer. She became the first human liver recipient with survival exceeding one year. Starzl knew he was on to something. In the next few years, he conducted as many as 175 liver transplants, experiencing a survival rate of 30 to 50 per cent. However, he could not keep up the percentage when, in 1981, he moved to the University of Pittsburgh, with all of his first four patients dying. It was time to delve deeper. One of the concerns and biggest barriers in the success of transplantation surgeries had always been the acceptance of the donor organ by the recipient's body and its immunological response. In this respect, his pioneering use of anti-rejection drugs proved to be a game changer.

He devised a technique of starting treatment before transplantation and adding anti-rejection drugs later, making Pittsburgh one of the busiest and most successful transplant centres in the world.

The list of awards and accolades gathered by him during the course of his career is endless, and include the National Medal of Science, David M. Hume Memorial Award, Benjamin Franklin Medal for Distinguished Achievement in the Sciences and the Lasker Award. He was also presented with honorary degrees by as many as 26 universities from various countries. In 1995, he was also honoured with the Grand-Cross of the Military Order of Saint James of the Sword, Portugal. The Pittsburgh Transplantation Institute, which was established in 1985, was renamed in 1996 as Thomas E. Starzl Transplantation Institute. One of the new medical research buildings in the University of Pittsburgh was named after him as the Thomas E. Starzl Biomedical Science Tower in 2006.

However, for someone who pioneered such challenging and crucial surgeries, Starzl never really enjoyed the process of surgery, as his contemporaries recall. Roy Calne, the UK surgeon who performed the first liver transplant in Europe in 1968, said, 'Tom may not have liked surgery, but he was very good at it.' He retired in 1991 from surgical practice but continued with his passion: research. He also taught at the University of Pittsburgh School of Medicine. After his death in 2017, a statue of Starzl was inaugurated on 24 June 2018 on the University of Pittsburgh campus.

[11] WIRGINIA MAIXNER

Wirginia Maixner's decision to study medicine came from two things she loved as a child – sewing and a television show about a doctor. Being a surgeon seemed to appear as a great way of combining these two things, she thought. She was also inspired by her aunt, who was Australia's first female flying doctor. Maixner is one of the few women in her field, paving the way forward in neurosurgery. While she spent a major part of her time working on children with epilepsy, she first hit the headlines in 2007 for performing the first auditory brainstem implant on a child in Australia. Two years later, she led a team of doctors as they successfully separated conjoined twins from Bangladesh.

Born in 1963, she grew up in Sydney and attended Sancta Sophia College, University of Sydney. In 1986, she graduated from the University of Sydney's School of Medicine with a Bachelor of Medicine, Bachelor of Surgery. She was only the third woman to be accepted into the Royal Australasian College of Surgeons four-year neurosurgery training program. 'Surgery at that stage was a difficult profession for women; it was a very male-dominated profession. Neurosurgery was one of the most challenging specialties, I think... Neurosurgery itself was still growing and paediatric neurosurgery was not quite as well established in some ways, certainly not as popular as many other things. So it was a bit unusual,' she is quoted to have said.

Part of Maixner's training was spent at The Royal Children's Hospital in Melbourne. While in the middle of the four-year training, she found herself unexpectedly pregnant. However, she decided to continue with the programme and became the first person to be granted maternity leave by the Royal Australasian College of Surgeons. Typically, during the early years of their career, surgeons were expected to work round the clock as it was perceived that non-stop, uninterrupted training was the best way to learn. After giving birth, she moved out of Australia with her newborn daughter as the training programme also required her to spend two years overseas in Canada and France. With her parents accompanying them, she gained international hospital experience as a single mother. She credits her parents for essentially giving up their own lives to be with her and take care of her daughter, especially at this crucial juncture in her career. In France, she had the incredible opportunity to train at the Necker-Enfants Malades in Paris, a paediatric neurosurgery hub that handled five times the cases that Melbourne did at the time.

The family returned to Melbourne and Maixner joined The Royal Children's Hospital in 1998. Around this time, she was doing both adult neurosurgery at The Royal Melbourne Hospital and paediatric neurosurgery at The Royal Children's Hospital. In 2001, she was appointed as head of department at The Royal Children's Hospital, becoming one of the first full-time paediatric neurosurgeons in Australia. She was also one of the youngest neurosurgery department heads in Australia. In 2006, Maixner performed path-breaking surgery on a three-year-old girl to successfully stop seizures caused due to a rare genetic condition. The next year, working in tandem with Rob Briggs, the medical director at the Royal Victorian Eye and Ear Hospital's Cochlear Implant Clinic, she used pioneering technology to achieve the first auditory brainstem implant on a child in Australia. The surgery was hailed as a breakthrough.

She gained international repute for her leading role in the series of surgeries to separate Bangladeshi conjoined twins Krishna and Trishna. A series of operations were performed in January, February, March, May, October and November 2008 and January and August 2009 to prepare for the final separation in November 2009. With a team of 16 doctors, including neurosurgeons, plastic surgeons, and other specialist medical staff at The Royal Children's Hospital, the final surgery was a 32-hour marathon to successfully separate the three-year-olds. The surgery put all eyes on Maixner. She, while acknowledging it would be a challenge, did not feel it would be the most difficult procedure of her life as the girls were already at death's door when she first met them, and she felt things could only get better from there.

Maixner continues to practice surgery and is a role model to women everywhere.

[12]
MICHAEL ELLIS DEBAKEY

A legendary surgeon, educator and innovator, Michael Ellis DeBakey's work transformed cardiovascular surgery, raised medical education standards and influenced national healthcare policy. A pioneer in surgical procedures for treatment of defects and diseases of the cardiovascular system, he worked on aneurysm repair, coronary bypass and endarterectomy. He also performed some of the first heart transplants and invented artificial hearts and ventricular assist pumps. He was an unstoppable force of nature, who, at the age of 97, underwent and recovered from a procedure he had pioneered 50 years earlier: the DeBakey procedure for aortic dissection.

He was born Michel Dabaghi in 1908 to Lebanese immigrants Shaker Morris and Raheeja Debaghi. His name was later Anglicized to Michael DeBakey. He grew up with three sisters and a brother – most of whom built careers in science – in Lake Charles, Louisiana. His interactions with doctors at his father's drugstore fanned his interest in medical science. After attending school in Lake Charles, he was off to New Orleans for his premedical course at Tulane University. In 1929, he began studying medicine at Tulane University School of Medicine. His spark of genius could be witnessed even before the completion of medical school as, in his final year, he devised a roller pump to facilitate blood transfusion continuously from one person to another. His invention would later become a vital part of the heart-lung machine. In 1932, he received his MD and stayed on in New Orleans for his internship and residency. Surgical fellowships took him to the University of Strasbourg, France and the University of Heidelberg, Germany. From 1942 to 1946, DeBakey served in the Second World War in the Surgical Consultants Division of the Army Surgeon General's Office. He returned to Tulane in 1946 to surgical practice and a teaching position at the university.

In 1948, he accepted a position as head of the department of surgery at Baylor University College of Medicine in Houston. It was not a big school at the time. Neither did it have a teaching hospital nor a clinical faculty. He worked tirelessly to start a surgical residency programme, revamped the medical curriculum, established surgical research labs, and raised money for the medical school. He also hired some staff and a faculty. According to the US National Library of Medicine, 'In 1952, he and Denton Cooley were the first Americans to successfully repair an abdominal aortic aneurysm, removing the weakened and distended section of the vessel and replacing it with a section of preserved cadaver aorta. (French surgeon Charles Dubost had done a similar operation the previous year.) They quickly applied the technique to progressively more difficult aneurysm repairs in the upper sections of the aorta. Within several years, they were fabricating the grafts from DuPont's new Dacron material, and DeBakey then helped design a special knitting machine to manufacture them.' In the 1950s, the first heart–lung bypass machines were fashioned and DeBakey and his team were the first ones to use them. 'DeBakey also devised techniques to repair dissecting aneurysms, and was the first to successfully perform procedures such as carotid endarterectomy and patch-graft angioplasty. In 1964 he did the first successful coronary bypass operation, and in 1968, the first multiple-organ transplant,' states documents at the library.

After 20 years at the institution, Baylor College of Medicine separated from Baylor University in 1968. DeBakey was at the helm of affairs, serving as CEO. Over the course of time, he rose to the position of chair of the department of surgery, serving until 1993. He continued to perform surgery till the age of 90 and was dubbed as the 'Texas Tornado' by cardiologist Paul Dudley White. He wrote more than 1,600 articles and performed over 60,000 surgeries. He won several awards and accolades during his career spanning 75 years. DeBakey passed away in 2008, at the age of 99, just two months short of his hundredth birthday.

[13]
PERCIVALL POTT

Percivall Pott, one of the founders of orthopaedics, was the first scientist to prove that cancer could occur due to an environmental carcinogen. He was renowned for his insightful and comprehensive surgical writings and honed the skills of several star surgeons, such as John Hunter. Pott was one of the first lecturers of anatomy elected by the Company of Surgeons, which is now the Royal College of Surgeons. His name is also listed in the *Annals of Medicine*.

Born in 1714 in London, Pott lost his father when he was very little and was mainly raised by his mother. After completing his schooling in a private school in Kent, he apprenticed under surgeon Edward Nourse at St. Bartholomew's Hospital in London. Pott would go on to have a long association with this iconic hospital. He was engaged in the dissection of cadavers for Nourse's anatomy classes, learning a great deal about surgery in the process. After spending seven years under Nourse, in 1736, Pott qualified for what is now the Royal College of Surgeons of England. Pott was honoured by being presented with the Grand Diploma in recognition for his outstanding surgical skills. He became an assistant surgeon at St. Bartholomew's in 1745 and was promoted to full surgeon after four years in 1749.

In his classic book *Chirurgical Observations Relative*

to the Cataract, the Polyplus of the Nose, the Cancer of the Scrotum, the Different Kinds of Ruptures, and the Mortification of the Toes and Feet, published in 1775, Pott first talked about cancer caused due to occupational exposure. Observing a rather high incidence of skin sores on the scrotums of men working as chimney sweeps, he also found soot deposits in the sores. He eventually concluded that men who were frequently exposed to soot were at a high risk for scrotal cancer. Pott's report was the first to pin down an environmental factor as a cause of cancer. The disease became known as chimney-sweepers' cancer. It later came to be known as testicular cancer. Pott's pivotal work made the medical fraternity aware of the concept of occupational medicine, leading the way for several groundbreaking studies on the subject. His research proved very valuable to the chimney sweeps' community as they could now steer clear of scrotal cancer by using protective clothing.

Another of Pott's significant contribution was clinically describing Pott disease – an ailment of the vertebrae in which the bones soften and collapse, making the spine curve, leading to a hunched back. It was caused due to arthritic tuberculosis of the spine. The Pott's fracture, which he sustained himself in 1756, was also named after him after he published a paper on its management. He described the fracture in 1768 as a fracture of the distal fibula, very close to the ankle joint. When he had sustained the fracture, doctors had discussed amputation – a very unrefined procedure at the time. However, after discussion with his mentor Nourse, Pott decided to splint the leg instead and recovered in a few months. His proposal for management of the fracture led to a decline in amputation rates for such fractures. He also described the Pott puffy tumour in 1768, a swelling of the scalp secondary to osteomyelitis of the skull as a complication of head trauma.

He passed away in 1788, after a rewarding and satisfying career.

[14]
LAWSON TAIT

Though gynaecology as a specialty flourished mainly in America, the Scottish surgeon Lawson Tait, who practiced in the late 19th century, made some major contributions to the field. He was widely known as the first to perform salpingectomy to treat a ruptured ectopic pregnancy. According to the February 2002 issue of the journal *Obstetrics and Gynecology*, 'he was also the first to record removal of an ovary for relief of pelvic pain and to induce menopause, perform salpingectomy for the treatment of tubal disease, and develop the technique of transverse transperineal repair of low rectovaginal fistulas.' He was known for his immaculate hygiene practices in the operation theatre. His innovative surgical techniques can be credited with a substantial decrease in surgical mortality, and led to several changes in the practice of obstetrics, resulting in a reduction in maternal morbidity and mortality. Tait was also an extraordinary educator and shaped the next great generation of abdominal and pelvic surgeons.

Born Robert Lawson Tait in Edinburgh in 1945, to lawyer Archibald Campbell Tait and Isabella Stewart Lawson, he was an exceptional student. At the age of 15, he won a scholarship to attend the University of Edinburgh as a student of arts, later changing his course in order to study medicine. In 1866, he graduated and received his Licentiate of the Royal College of Physicians. He then worked at the Clayton Hospital in Wakefield as a resident surgeon for four years, where he made bold advances in surgery in the abdomen and even performed an ovariotomy. In 1870, he switched to private practice in Birmingham, England, where he also became a member of the British Medical Association. Later, he also pursued a fellowship at the Obstetrical Society of London as he wanted to establish himself as an integral part of his new city.

His pioneering career included several firsts such as the first removal of an organ (ovary) for pain and the first cholecystotomy (gall bladder surgery). He also conducted what was at that time known as the first appendectomy. However, it was later revealed that a French-born English surgeon had preceded him, as early as 1735. Some of his other surgical milestones were observing the link between cystic ovaries and excessive menstrual bleeding, the surgical induction of menopause through the removal of ovaries, surgical removal of infected tubes, and drainage of pelvic abscess. He also emerged as a champion in the management of ectopic pregnancies, a condition that had previously been life-threatening. He began the surgical removal of ruptured fallopian tubes after observing a post-mortem in 1881. By 1888, Tait had operated on 42 patients – with only two deaths. Much of his surgical success can be attributed to the introduction of asepsis practices in his operations. Tait and Joseph Lister were both strong advocates of reducing the chances of infection by cleaning hands and instruments. While Lister advocated antisepsis by sterilization with chemicals, Tait simply used boiling water to sterilize instruments. He achieved good results with this simple, effective, and economical approach.

Tait wholeheartedly supported Arthur Chamberlain in his endeavour of developing a hospital that would cater exclusively to women and their conditions. The duo were successful in establishing the hospital and Tait continued to work there for a long time. For his advocacy of new techniques and pro-vivisection arguments, Tait was seen by many as a controversial figure. However, to his students, he was exemplary. He passed away in 1899 at the age of 54, after suffering from chronic nephritis and uremia. The Lawson Tait Society, an undergraduate society that focuses on the history of medicine, was established to honour him at the University of Birmingham Medical School.

[15]
SIR HENRY SOUTTAR

Sir Henry Souttar's obituary in the *British Heart Journal* described him as a 'distinguished and daring surgeon'. Souttar was also a multitasker with a wide range of interests, which converged brilliantly to help him advance in his career. An engineer with a penchant for mathematics and medicine, he was able to combine his knowledge of the three to invent various innovative surgical instruments. He was responsible for drafting the first British guidelines for radiotherapy. However, his best-known achievement was performing the first ever trans-auricular mitral valvotomy in 1925. It was the first intracardiac handling of the living human heart by the human hand on a patient with a congenital heart defect – sort of like an open-heart surgery performed while blindfolded. It was something that wouldn't be repeated for years.

Souttar was born in Birkenhead in Merseyside, England in 1875 to Robinson and Mary Souttar. His father was an engineer and later Member of Parliament for Dumfries. After completing his schooling in Oxford High School, he went on to gain a 'Double First', or two first-class honours, in mathematics and also study engineering at Queen's College in Oxford. He was also an exceptional athlete who was very fond of rowing and continued to indulge in it well over the age of 60. His mathematical and engineering training made him older than most of the other students when he qualified for Bachelor of Medicine and BCh in 1906. He went on to work at London Hospital and became a fellow of the Royal College of Surgeons in 1909. In 1914, during the First World War, he went to Antwerp and was part of the dangerous and exhausting evacuation to Furnes, near the front line when the battle raged round the Ypres Salient. An account of his experience took the shape of the book *A Surgeon in Belgium*. He also served as the chief surgeon to the British Red Cross Hospital at Netley. Once the war was through, he resumed his duties at the London Hospital. In 1920, he was made the director of the new surgical unit at the hospital, and thus began the most eventful time in his career.

The year was 1925 and surgery of the chest was in its nascent stages; operations on the valves of the heart were unheard of. Souttar operated on a patient with mitral valve disease, devising a new procedure, which proved to be a success. According to the *British Heart Journal*, 'He decided there was no need to increase the mitral opening which admitted his finger, and was content to break down the adhesions that tethered down the cusps. His patient, a girl aged 15, lived for seven years and was one of the only two who survived these early attempts.

It is surprising that Souttar was not asked to operate on others: he had done all that was then possible, but there was no great improvement and the physicians concerned did not recognize this was because the patient had preponderant mitral regurgitation.' Souttar's physician colleagues came to the conclusion that the procedure was not justified and so he could not continue. It was only in 1948 that something like this was attempted again. Nonetheless, he was the first surgeon to explore a valve with his finger.

Souttar used his profound knowledge of physics, engineering, and medicine to come up with a gun that could plant radon seeds around a tumour to treat it. He enjoyed a long career as an educator as well and wrote books such as *Injuries of the Peripheral Nerves*, *The Art of Surgery*, *Radium and its Surgical Applications*, and *Radium and Cancer*. He was a Bradshaw lecturer in 1943, Hunterian orator in 1949, and served as the president of the British Medical Association in 1945–46. He was knighted in 1949. Years after his pioneering operation, he was made an Honorary Member of the British Cardiac Society.

Souttar died in 1964, a couple of years after the death of his first wife Catharine Edith in 1959. They were married for 55 years and he had a son and a daughter with her. He had remarried a widow, their family friend Amy Wigdahl, in 1963.

[16]
NITA AHUJA

A surgical leader and surgeon-scientist of international repute, Nita Ahuja is the first woman to serve as Chair of Surgery in Yale in its more than 200-year-old history. She is also the first woman to have been appointed Chief of Surgical Oncology at Johns Hopkins Hospital. The Indian-born American surgeon is known for her efficient handling of gastrointestinal cancer cases and performing complex surgeries for patients with gastric, rectal, and pancreatic cancers. Using minimally invasive surgical procedures, she has carved a niche for herself in treating rare, difficult soft-tissue sarcomas that affect the connective tissue.

Born in India, Ahuja moved to America as a young girl when her parents migrated. She always had a deep interest in science and began her career as a laboratory technician in the department of immunology, National Institutes of Health in Bethesda, Maryland. With research being her strong forte, she was awarded with the Outstanding College Students of America and Alpha Omega Alpha Original Research Award for her extraordinary research work. She studied medicine at Duke University in Durham, North Carolina, followed by a fellowship in surgical oncology at Johns Hopkins Hospital in Baltimore, USA. While conducting her postdoctoral research, she first talked about the notion of

CpG Island Methylator Phenotype (CIMP) or CpG island hypermethylation in colorectal cancer. This concept of CIMP has now been identified to have implications for prognosis and response to therapy. It has been proven to occur in multiple other tumour types such as glioblastomas, leukaemia, duodenal cancers, and more.

Ahuja is an exceptional researcher whose studies have been cited as many as 11,000 times and counting. The National Institutes of Health-funded surgeon-scientist is also a leading member of the second Stand Up to Cancer Dream Team since 2008, a research group involved in reviewing epigenetic therapy for cancer management. Over the years, she has emerged as a trailblazer in translational epigenetics, and has been organizing clinical trials in colorectal cancer, pancreatic cancer, and other solid tumours. Another one of her significant achievements has been the development of biomarkers for the timely discovery of colorectal and pancreatic cancers. Ahuja has led more than 20 national and international clinical trials that have tested novel therapies in gastrointestinal and breast cancers based on theories identified in her laboratory. She believes in working with a variety of treatment modalities to deliver the most effective results and has especially excelled in management of peritoneal cancer metastases with cytoreduction and heated intraperitoneal chemotherapy.

Ahuja is a part of several prestigious medical associations and groups such as the National Academy of

Medicine, American Surgical Association, New England Surgical Society, Southern Surgical Association, and the Association of American Medical Colleges Council of Faculty and Academic Societies Administrative Board. The awards and honours in she has received include the William J. Reinhoff Jr. Scholar Award, the American Surgical Association Fellowship, the Society of Surgical Oncology Clinical Investigator Award, and the Abell Foundation Award: Johns Hopkins Alliance for Science and Technology Development. She has also won the Exceptional Women in Medicine Award in 2017 and 2019.

Since February 2018, she has been at the helm of affairs as chair of the department of surgery at Yale School of Medicine and chief of surgery at the Yale New Haven Hospital.

[17]
BENJAMIN S. CARSON, SR.

Before retiring and turning to politics, Benjamin S. Carson, Sr. made some waves in the operating theatre. At the young age of 33, he was the youngest person in the history of the John Hopkins Children's Center to be appointed as the Director of Pediatric Neurosurgery. He hit the limelight when he successfully separated occipital craniopagus twins conjoined at the back of the head in 1987. He was also roped in for the first fully successful separation of type-2 vertical craniopagus twins in South Africa a few years later. Carson also further fine-tuned a surgical technique known as hemispherectomy, which involves the removal of one-half of the brain to control seizures in patients suffering from severe epilepsy. He was also the first to come up with an intra-uterine procedure to relieve pressure on the brain of a hydrocephalic foetal twin.

Born in 1951 in Detroit, Michigan, Carson was a below-average student during his early years. His parents, Robert Solomon Carson Jr. – who was a World War II veteran – and Sonya Carson, divorced when Carson was just eight years old. Thereafter, he lived with his mother, who worked two to three jobs to make ends meet, and his older brother, Curtis. With some interventions by his mother, the academic performance of both the brothers improved and Carson developed a new-found interest to learn. For his college education, Carson applied at Yale and was accepted, receiving a full scholarship. He graduated with a BA in psychology in 1973. His next stop was the University of Michigan, where he earned a medical degree in 1977. Carson completed a residency in neurosurgery after that at Johns Hopkins University Medical School. In 1984, he became the director of paediatric neurosurgery at Johns Hopkins, becoming one of the youngest doctors in the country to rise to such a position.

The year 1987 came with the biggest challenge for

Carson: the case of German twins conjoined at the head. He was only 35 at the time and had offered the scalpel to his boss Donlin Long, who was the head of neurosurgery at Johns Hopkins. Long refused, and it was all in Carson's young hands. No twins conjoined at the head had ever been separated successfully and there were no reference points for him. He decided to use a radical approach wherein the body temperatures of the patients would be lowered to the point of circulatory arrest. It had its risks but there were hardly any other options. It took a team of 70 doctors and medical staff and 28 hours to separate them. According to a report in the *Washington Post*, 'For four hours, heart surgeons inserted "hair-thin" tubes into their veins and connected them to heart-lung machines that would keep them alive through surgery. Plastic surgeons sliced into their scalp, removing the bone tissue that connected them. The cardiologists then cut open their chests and removed small amounts of tissue from their heart to use later to construct new veins.' At last, it was done. The planning and subsequent success of the procedure as well as the reconstructive techniques used made Carson an overnight sensation. He became the subject of a 2009 television film *Gifted Hands: The Ben Carson Story*. However, while this was the first time twins conjoined at the head had been separated with success, they had to live with neurologic and medical complications.

The list of awards and honours bestowed upon Carson

are exhausting. Some of the most noteworthy ones are the Presidential Medal of Freedom, the nation's highest civilian honour, and the Spingarn Medal, the highest honor bestowed by the National Association for the Advancement of Colored People (NAACP).

By the time he retired in 2013, he was professor of neurosurgery, oncology, plastic surgery, and paediatrics at the Johns Hopkins School of Medicine. He had published several books and countless papers. After a rewarding career in surgery, he joined politics full time, even participating in the 2016 presidential run. He also served as the US Secretary of Housing and Urban Development from 2017 to 2021.

[18]
CHRISTIAAN BARNARD

A keen observer who wasn't afraid to take risks, Christiaan Barnard had all the trappings of a pioneering surgeon who had the guts to attempt the first human-to-human heart transplant. He was only a resident surgeon at Cape Town's Groote Schurr Hospital when he illustrated that intestinal atresia, a congenital opening in the small intestine, is caused by insufficient blood supply to the foetus in the mother's womb, leading to the development of a surgical way to fix the fatal defect. The cardiothoracic surgeon also introduced open-heart surgery in his country.

Born in 1922 at Beaufort West, Cape Province, in South Africa, he was the third of four sons to Adam and Maria Barnard. One of his siblings was a blue baby and died of a congenital heart defect at the age of three. This could have inspired Barnard's interest in the human heart. He began studying medicine at the University of Cape Town's Medical School in 1940. After a couple of years interning and working in some hospitals in South Africa, he was offered a scholarship at the University of Minnesota in 1956. Belonging to a family of limited means, it was an incredible opportunity for the young doctor to be under the wing of renowned Professor Owen Wangensteen. This was his first brush with the new field of open-heart surgery, though he was assigned to work on the intestines. The university hospital in Minneapolis was one of the few in the world where this form of surgery was being conducted. Barnard was impressed with what he saw and felt there was great potential in the heart-lung machine.

Upon returning to South Africa in 1958, he was appointed head of the department of experimental surgery at Groote Schuur Hospital and also taught at the University of Cape Town. In 1967, he conducted the first ever human-to-human heart transplant. According to *Global Cardiology Science and Practice*, 'The daring operation and the charismatic surgeon received immense public attention around the world. The patient's progress was covered by the world's media on an almost hourly basis.' Unfortunately, the 54-year-old patient, Louis Washansky, never left the hospital and died after only 18 days after contracting double pneumonia. With anti-rejection drugs playing a role in suppressing immune function, recovery was difficult. 'Barnard soon carried out a second transplant, and this patient led an active life for almost 19 months. Remarkably, Barnard's fifth and sixth patients lived for almost 13 and 24 years, respectively. Barnard subsequently introduced the operation of heterotopic heart transplantation in which the donor heart acted as an auxiliary pump, with some advantages in that early era. It took great courage to carry out the first heart transplant, and this is why Barnard is remembered as a pioneer in cardiac surgery.'

Soon after the procedure, the trend of experimenting with heart transplants spread like wildfire. Surgeons in as many as 24 countries began toying with the procedure, many with no relevant experience with the concept. With low rates of success, heart transplants began dwindling around the world. However, Barnard kept at it and, to a great degree, perfected the technique in the 1970s. Barnard served as the head of the cardiac unit at Groote Schuur Hospital until 1983. Unfortunately, he was forced to retire as a surgeon when he began suffering from rheumatoid arthritis in his hands. However, he remained active with research and was engaged with several institutions. He died in 2001 while on holiday in Cyprus, when he suffered an acute asthma attack.

[19]
FERDINAND ADOLF KEHRER

A German gynaecologist, Ferdinand Adolf Kehrer is widely regarded as the father of the modern caesarean section (C-section). The transverse technique which minimized bleeding when performing a C-section, was introduced by Kehrer. Caesarean sections at the time were still risky procedures due to the rudimentary techniques employed during the surgery, low standards of clinical practices, and general hygiene. Symphysiotomy, a procedure in which the cartilage of the pubic symphysis is divided to widen the pelvis, prevailed before C-sections gained popularity gradually and emerged as a safer and more viable option. According to the *International Journal of Applied and Basic Medical Research,* the 'history of cesarean section in India dates back to 320 BC when Chanakya, the great Indian emperor, Chandragupta's teacher, and advisor, cut open the belly of the queen and took out the baby, thus saving his life, when the queen died accidently after consuming poison. Initially, cesarean section resulted in death of the mother. The first well-recorded incident of a woman surviving cesarean section was in 1580 in Switzerland.' The status of the C-section as a commonplace procedure today can largely be traced back to the surgery conducted by Kehrer in 1881.

Born in 1837, Kehrer was a native of Guntersblum in Rhenish Hesse. After completing his medical studies at the University of Giessen under Ferdinand von Ritgen, Karl von Hecker and Karl von Braun-Fernwald, he served as professor of obstetrics at the university. He began to work as director of the University Women's Clinic in Heidelberg from 1881, when he relocated to the University of Heidelberg as Chair of Gynaecology. It was in Heidelberg that he performed the first conservative classical C-section. The patient, Emelie Schussler, was a 28-year-old woman from Meckesheim. The uterus was not cut open from top to bottom, as was standard practice until then, but across at the lower segment of the uterus. It is said that Kehrer used this surgical method for the first time in Schussler's house in Meckesheim, which is still preserved and is open to visitors. The entire procedure took about one hour, with the mother and child both responding well and surviving into old age without any complications. Before Kehrer's novel technique, the maternal mortality rate associated with C-sections was 80 per cent. With his method, it was lowered down to a negligible 0.1 per cent.

The professor's success laid the foundation for future advancements in the procedure. In the years to come, uterine suturing was introduced by fellow German gynaecologist Max Saenger in 1882. Yet another German gynaecologist, Hermann Johannes Pfannenstiel, modified the incision used by Kehrer, which was again altered in 1912. It is still one of the most widely used techniques for the procedure. These medical breakthroughs and innovations, complemented by the advances in anaesthesia, blood transfusion, antibiotics, and the standards of asepsis, led to the popularity of the C-section.

Kehrer also wrote a textbook for midwives and another one on obstetrics, as well as publishing several papers. He died in Heidelberg in 1914.

[20]
IOANNIS PALLIKARIS

Ioannis Pallikaris is a name to reckon with in his field and was the man behind LASIK, or laser-eye surgery for the correction of refractive conditions such as myopia. He was the first to use the LASIK technique on a human eye. He later also developed Epi-LASIK and described the Photoablatable Lenticular Modulator (PALM) technique for corneal resurfacing. He was one of the inventors of the Tracey ray-tracing device for clinical aberrometry. Apart from being a game changer in ophthalmology, Palikaris is an excellent educator and has been teaching for over 30 years in Greece and Switzerland at undergraduate and post-graduate levels.

Born in 1847, in Chania, in the island of Crete in Greece, Pallikaris obtained his medical degree from the Aristotle University of Thessaloniki, Greece, in 1972. For his residency and PhD thesis, he was off to the University of Zurich, Switzerland in 1981, where he trained under Professor Rudolf Witmer. After being trained in the anterior segment, Pallikaris eventually trained as a vitreo-retina surgeon. After his stint in Zurich, he returned to Crete in the late 1980s. His extensive training made him an easychoice for the position of the Director of the department of ophthalmology at the University of Crete. Refractive surgery was of great interest to him, and once back on his home turf, he began focusing on it. At the University of Crete he founded the Institute of Vision and Optics (IVO), which would become the first place in the world where the first LASIK surgery would be performed in 1989. 'Since then, he had a great impact in the field of ophthalmology... he is considered "the father of LASIK," the most worldwide acknowledged and used surgical technique in correcting refractive errors, at present. For patients, LASIK became synonymous with refractive surgery similar to XEROX is to photocopy,' states a 2020 article in the *Indian Journal of Opthalmology*.

Palikaris was the Rector of the University of Crete between 2003 and 2011. He serves as the Medical Advisory Board Chair for ophthalmic device company Presbia, where he is responsible for a corneal inlay treatment for presbyopia. He also conducts training sessions for surgeons at the Vardinoyannion Eye Institute of Crete.

According to the article in the *Indian Journal of*

Opthalmology, 'Another significant invention of Prof Pallikaris is ray tracing technology, to track the optics of the human eye, which he started studying in 1992. Further, The TRACEY device, developed in collaboration with the Kiev Institute of Biomedical Technology (Ukraine) was one of the first commercial instruments for the measurement of the optical aberrations of the human eye and the assessment of retinal image quality. He also developed a rotating brush to remove the epithelium: it is a very practical innovation and many of us use it during the surface ablation procedure. Around 2000, Professor Pallikaris developed Epi-LASIK, a very popular technique of surface ablation for patients with thin corneas. All microkeratome manufacturers quickly adapted to Epi-LASIK and it became one of the preferred choices for surface ablation.'

The author of several opthalmology textbooks, he can boast of 200 articles that have been published in international journals. He also holds over 20 patents related to optics and ophthalmology. Palikaris has been the proud recipient of various awards such as the AAO Lifetime Achievement Award and the ESCRS (European Society of Cataract and Refractive Surgery) Binkhorst Medal. In 2005, he became the vice president of the National Council for Research and Technology, and the next year, he became a member of the Plenum of the Greek National Committee for UNESCO. He was elected President of the European Society of Cataract and

Refractive Surgery (ESCRS) and served in the position from 2006 to 2008. Apart from his work on LASIK and similar treatments, he is known for his research on corneal and iris biology, ocular imaging, corneal implants and inlays, and corneal collagen cross-linking.

TWO

THOSE WHO KEEP THE TICKER TICKING

SINCE THE ERA OF THE INTRODUCTION OF electrocardiography in 1902, to the advent of external pacemakers 50 years later and the more recent transcatheter aortic valve implantation in 2002, heart surgery has come a long way. The leaps and bounds of progress have certainly taken years of research, determination, and hard work by researchers and surgeons. Technology, too, has lent a helping hand in the process of modernizing the care of the human heart. Ailments of the heart are rising and are among the leading causes of death in people, making the role of heart surgeons and doctors more relevant than ever.

From adopting some of the world's latest systems and technologies to building upon age-old techniques and innovating out-of-the-box surgeries, these are the surgeons who have changed the face of heart surgery.

[1]
DENTON COOLEY

The founder of the Texas Heart Institute, Denton Cooley is the surgeon behind several of today's frequently used cardiovascular procedures and devices. In 1968, he became the first person to transplant a human heart successfully in the United States. He was also the first to implant mechanical devices like the total artificial heart and left ventricular assist device, and undertook the first successful carotid endarterectomy. He fashioned techniques for repairing diseased heart valves, congenital cardiac anomalies, and aortic and ventricular aneurysms. At a time when open-heart surgery was in its nascent stages and surgeons would only do two procedures per day, Cooley, employing his innovative approach, would manage a dozen.

Born in Houston, Texas, in 1920, Cooley followed in the footsteps of his father, who was a dentist, and his maternal grandfather, who was a physician. Interestingly, he attended the University of Texas as a pre-dental student and it was on a dare that he visited an emergency room for the first time. After suturing his first lacerations there, he switched to pre-medical. After graduating in 1941 from the University of Texas at Austin, he completed his medical degree and surgical training at the Johns Hopkins School of Medicine in Baltimore, Maryland. During his internship at Johns Hopkins, he got the opportunity to work with legendary surgeon Alfred Blalock and even assisted him in the first blue baby procedure to correct an infant's congenital heart defect.

After a couple of years serving in the Army Medical Corps in Austria, he began working with renowned British surgeon Russell Brock at the Royal Brompton Hospital in London in 1950. A couple of years later, he returned to Houston, becoming associate professor of surgery at Baylor College of Medicine. Here, he began working with the legendary Michael DeBakey. Their association would eventually result in a long-standing professional rivalry, with Cooley resigning his position in 1969. The same year, he became the first to implant an artificial heart in a patient who lived for nearly three days after the procedure. In 1970, he became the first to implant an artificial heart in a human when no heart replacement was immediately available. He had already established himself as a skilled surgeon by performing various bloodless open-heart surgeries. By the end of his career, he had repaired as many as 12,000 aortic aneurysms.

With 12 books that bear his name, Cooley has authored or co-authored more than 1,300 papers. He was a member of more than 70 prestigious professional societies. The Texas Heart Institute made him an honorary member of the Denton A. Cooley Cardiovascular Surgical Society, which has been named after him. He has been the proud recipient of countless honours and awards including the National Medal of Technology and

Innovation, the Rene Leriche Prize, the Distinguished Service Award of the American Medical Association, the Gifted Teacher Award of the American College of Cardiology, and the Grand Hamdan International Award for Medical Science. While presenting him with the Presidential Medal of Freedom, the highest US civilian award, President Ronald Reagan lauded him, saying that Cooley 'has charted new territory in his search for ways to prolong and enrich human life'.

Cooley passed away in 2016, at the age of 96.

[2]
RUSSELL M. NELSON

A heart surgeon-turned-apostle, Russell M. Nelson had a long and eventful medical career before switching to religious duties. He always thought of his medical practice as an expression of his faith, a way to serve others. Born in 1924 in Salt Lake City, Utah, Nelson had a perfect pitch and grew up singing in the church choir. He graduated from the University of Utah in 1945, earning his medical degree in 1947. For his postdoctoral studies, he was off to the University of Minnesota.

Nelson's most valuable contribution to heart surgery came when he, along with his colleagues, invented the first heart–lung machine. After its development in the early 1950s, it opened up a 'new world' for heart surgery, according to the surgeon. The machine made the world's first open-heart surgical procedure possible in 1951. In 1955, upon his return to his home state, he became the first surgeon to perform open-heart surgery in Utah, using his own heart-lung machine. He also worked as a surgeon at Latter Day Saints Hospital, which was a long and fruitful union. Along with this, Nelson served as a faculty member in surgery and as the director of the Thoracic Surgery Residency Program at the University of Utah School of Medicine. He worked there tirelessly for nearly two decades, improving upon several cardiovascular surgery techniques and grooming generations of cardiac surgeons.

He was a celebrated surgeon, and his knack for coming up with innovative heart procedures made him the clear choice to operate on the then-LDS (The Church of Jesus Christ of Latter-day Saints) president Spencer Kimball and Chinese performer Fang Rongxiang. He earned several awards and accolades and held several positions of authority, such as the President of the Thoracic Surgical Directors Association, President of the Society for Vascular Surgery, President of the Utah State Medical Association, and Director of the American Board of Thoracic Surgery. The American Heart Association presented him with the Heart of Gold Award, while the American Academy of Achievement awarded him the Golden Plate Award. He also earned the Governor's Medal of Science: Lifetime Achievement Award at the Utah Technology Innovation Summit.

Just when he was at the height of his surgical career, he was called to be an apostle in 1984. Today, he is a high-ranking leader of the Mormon faith. At 96 years of age, he serves as the President of the LDS Church.

[3]
RAMAKANTA PANDA

Regarded as one of the finest cardiac surgeons in the world, Ramakanta Panda grew from humble beginnings in a small village in Odisha, India. With a 99.7 per cent success rate in bypass surgery, he has emerged as one of the safest heart surgeons in the world. He has performed surgeries on various eminent political figures such as Manmohan Singh when he was serving as Prime Minister, and several heads of states, like Lalu Prasad Yadav and the late Tarun Gogoi. He is regarded as the pioneer of 'off-pump' bypass surgery, which is performed on a beating heart. He was also one the first few surgeons in the country to introduce the concept of total arterial revascularization, in which an artery from the patient's leg or wrist is grafted to the coronary arteries in order to bypass the blocked portions.

Born in 1954 in Damodarpur, Panda studied for two years at BJB College before switching to Sriram Chandra Bhanja Medical College in Cuttack. Thereafter, he trained in cardiac surgery from the All India Institute of Medical Sciences (AIIMS), New Delhi, where he was a topper.

He then flew to the US for his fellowship training at Cleveland Clinic, under surgeon Floyd Loop, a pioneer of bypass surgery. He also briefly trained under Denton Cooley (whose record of number of surgeries Panda may break soon) during the eight years he was in America. He then spent two years as an associate staff senior registrar at the Harefield Hospital in the UK, training under the legendary Professor Magdi Yacoub.

Back in India in 1993, Panda was yearning to open a world-class hospital. 'I really had that burning desire to come back to India and build a hospital that would rank among the best in the world. It took me seven years,' he said in an interview. His dream materialized at the Bandra-Kurla Complex (BKC) in Mumbai in 2000. While OPD services were inaugurated at the Asian Heart Institute in 2002, surgeries began in early 2003. In just a few years, the Asian Heart Institute has emerged as a benchmark hospital, with a lot of firsts to its credit, such as jointless flooring, a special ICU, hand washbasins for every ICU bed and counselling rooms for family members of patients.

At his award-winning hospital, Panda has performed some breakthrough surgeries. He fixed 17 blocks in the heart of a patient using a record number of 12 grafts to restore blood flow. Another patient suffering from an extremely rare heart condition, with a risk of developing permanent infections, was also treated by Panda. The 39-year-old's heart valve was successfully repaired with a first-of-its-kind surgery. He also performed a six-hour surgery to remove a rare heart tumour, in addition to fixing three blocks on a 62-year-old patient.

Panda has set up two charitable trusts to help economically challenged patients while continuing to work at the Asian Heart Institute. He was honoured with the Padma Bhushan, India's third highest civilian award, in 2010.

[4]
RANDAS BATISTA

Randas Batista is credited with developing several revolutionary techniques – the Batista Procedure, in particular, earned him a lot of fame after initial scepticism. It entails removing a piece of the dilated heart (partial left ventriculectomy) to treat end-stage heart failure patients, eliminating the need of a transplant. Flouting the long-standing conventional idea of preserving heart tissue at all costs, Randas Batista cuts out large segments of enlarged hearts. The result is a smaller heart that is able to pump blood much more efficiently and has patients walking only two days after the surgery.

Born in 1947, Batista graduated from medical school in Curitiba, Brazil, in 1972. Thereafter, he spent 12 years in the United States, Canada, and Europe in surgical training. In 1983, he finally returned back home, to Campina Grande do Sul, a suburban village close to Curitiba.

His heart reduction surgery was met with a lot of raised eyebrows at first, probably because the surgical technique came from an unknown surgeon at a nondescript 200-bed hospital in a small Brazilian village. There was rejection and ridicule in store for him when he first discussed the idea at a medical conference in Boston in 1994. With nearly 70 per cent of patients with enlarged hearts requiring heart transplants, the ratio with donor hearts has always been quite mismatched. The Batista Procedure could take care of that without the hassle of a heart transplant and the risk of rejection by the recipient's body. Batista's approach, based on his observation of animal hearts, was simple – no matter what the size of an animal, the ratio of its heart's mass to its volume remains the same. Essentially, what that meant was that a bigger heart needs more muscle to pump blood efficiently. If the heart's radius doubles, eight times more muscle was required to pump blood well enough.

Cutting out a large slice of living muscle from the main pumping chamber of the heart, which is then stitched together when the heart is still beating, could help solve the problem. The blood would pump effectively. Slowly but surely, Batista's technique gained popularity as the results were promising. Several cardiac surgeons from Western countries would visit him in his humble hospital to learn the procedure that could be performed on a patient of any age. Batista also travelled extensively to developing nations, where his techniques were most required as they were cheap, effective, and fast. Most surgeries would only take about an hour. Though sophisticated techniques have replaced the Batista Procedure in several First World countries, it is still of great use in developing nations.

For his innovative and insightful technique, he earned several awards and accolades in several European countries and the United States. He was listed as one of the 15 world heroes of medicine in a list by *Time* magazine and CNN in 2012. His name has been engraved on a memorial on the island of Kos in Greece that honours the father of medicine, Hippocrates.

[5]
WILLIAM DEVRIES

William DeVries shot to fame when he performed the first artificial heart transplant on a human patient at the University of Utah Medical Center. He, along with his team, made medical history in 1982, when they replaced the diseased heart of a patient with the Jarvik-7, the first permanent artificial heart to be used in a human patient. DeVries was the only surgeon who had approval by the federal Food and Drug Administration (FDA) to implant an artificial heart into a human.

DeVries was born in 1943 in Brooklyn Navy Yard. His Dutch immigrant father, who was a physician in the navy, died in combat when he was a six-month-old baby. He was then brought up by his grandmother and his mother, who remarried and moved the family to Ogden, Utah. Though he had a mechanical inclination, he also excelled in sports and academics. In 1966, he passed out from the University of Utah with a bachelor's degree in molecular and genetic biology. He continued medical school at the University of Utah and received his MD in 1970. While in his first year of medical school, he attended a lecture by Dutch-born Willem Kolff, a pioneer of biomedical engineering. Impressed with his work, DeVries asked him for a position on his research team and got the chance to conduct experimental surgery on the first animal recipients of the artificial heart. For his internship and residency in cardiovascular surgery, the young doctor left for Duke University, eventually returning to Kolff's team in 1979.

This was the time when synthetic materials were being developed at a great pace and this boosted the development of permanent artificial hearts and other such devices. Designed by American physician Robert K. Jarvik, the Jarvik-7 was an aluminum and plastic device named after its inventor, which could replace two ventricles of the patient's heart. Two rubber diaphragms would mimic the pumping action of the biological heart. They were kept beating by an external compressor connected to the implant by pipes. After DeVries performed the surgery, the first recipient survived 112 days, eventually succumbing to some physical complications due to the implant.

The second implantation of Jarvik-7 happened at Louisville, Kentucky, where DeVries had newly joined at the Humana Heart Institute International. This patient suffered setbacks as well and the surgery was covered extensively by the media. After facing criticism, DeVries stated, 'People always look at artificial hearts as innovative therapy. But the other part is hard-core experimentation. You may exchange one set of complications for another.' Interestingly, the daring doctor attended the funerals of several of his patients, flouting standard practice. He even gave the eulogy at the funeral of one of his patients, at his widow's request. Five years since the first implantation, 49 Jarvik-7 hearts were implanted by several surgeons in different parts of the world. They especially proved to be useful in dying patients awaiting a human heart transplant. However, it didn't offer a long-term solution. In 1988, just as DeVries was about to perform his fifth Jarvik-7 transplant, a human donor heart was found for the patient. Two years later in 1990, the FDA withdrew its approval of the Jarvik-7, marking the end of the innovative programme.

A fellow of the American College of Cardiology and the American College of Surgeons, DeVries is also a member at both the institutions. After an eventful career in cardiac surgery, at the age of 58, he joined the staff at Walter Reed Army Medical Center as a Defense Department contractor and also joined the Army Reserve.

[6]
ANDREAS ROLAND GRÜNTZIG

An unusual combination of radiologist and cardiologist, Andreas Roland Grüntzig was the first to develop successful balloon angioplasty for expanding lumens of narrowed arteries. After gaining exposure to the Dotter technique (catheter-based dilation of peripheral arterial stenosis) in 1971, the idea for a balloon catheter took root in his mind. The German surgeon received no backing or funds for his venture. Neither the federal funding agencies nor the hospital where he was working approved of his ideas. However, he persevered, and with some help from his team, emerged successful in his experiments in 1973 and performed the procedure for the first time in 1974.

Born in Dresden, East Germany, in 1939 to Wilmar Grüntzig, who was a PhD in chemistry – as well as a writer, composer, and science teacher – and Charlotta Zeugner Grüntzig, who was a piano teacher, Grüntzig always showed a lot of promise as a student. He graduated with the highest honours from the Thomas Schule in Leipzig. Just before the Communist DDR government closed East Germany's borders, he made an exit to join his brother Johannes in Heidelberg, where he received his medical degree at Heidelberg University in 1964. He then interned in various specialties. But it was at the Max Ratschow Klinik in Darmstadt that he got the chance to perform his first peripheral artery angiographies. In 1969, he got a job at the University Hospital in Zurich, Switzerland, with renowned internal medicine specialist Robert Hegglin.

In 1971 in Engelskirchen, Eberhard Zeitler introduced him to the Dotter technique. Grüntzig was immediately fascinated and started working on a balloon catheter. Without any funding or support, he worked on it relentlessly over a span of two years with the support of his fiancée Michaela, Maria Schlumpf, his research assistant, and her engineer husband, Walter. Together, they innovated on a functional, handmade balloon catheter. In 1973, he moved to the Division of Cardiology of the Medical Policlinic of the University of Zurich, where he performed several angioplasty procedures using the Dotter technique. In February 1974, he performed the first peripheral angioplasty using his new single-lumen dilatation catheter with a 4-mm balloon on a patient suffering from incapacitating claudication due to a serious femoral artery stenosis. The next month, Grüntzig performed the first balloon angioplasty of an iliac artery stenosis. He published his findings with Heinrich Hopff, an emeritus professor of organic chemistry at the Federal Institute of Technology (ETH) in Zurich, based on the treatment of 15 patients on whom balloon angioplasty had been conducted. The Grüntzig balloon angioplasty procedure came to be known as 'percutaneous transluminal angioplasty,' or PTA, and he filed for patents on the concept in the USA, Switzerland,

Germany, France, England, and Japan. The procedure today is also known as Percutaneous Transluminal Coronary Angioplasty (PTCA) or Percutaneous Coronary Intervention (PCI) in coronary arteries. It is widely regarded as the method of choice to treat patients with acute myocardial infarction or occluded leg arteries.

At the young age of 46, Grüntzig and his wife passed away rather unfortunately in an airplane crash in 1985. He left behind a great legacy and an unfinished autobiography.

[7]
WILFRED C. BIGELOW

In 1950, Wilfred C. Bigelow had learnt how to how to lower the body's oxygen requirements while lowering its core temperature. His discovery first found practical use in 1953. He also pioneered another major advance in cardiac care – the pacemaker – that stemmed quite out of the blue from his hypothermia research in 1951. His discoveries and their practical implementation changed cardiac surgery for the better and helped millions of people suffering from heart disease. He also played a pivotal role in shaping the first formal cardiac surgery training programme in Canada.

Bigelow was born in 1913 in Brandon, Manitoba, Canada. His father, Wilfred Abram Bigelow, was a doctor and the founder of the first private medical clinic in Canada. His mother, Grace Ann Gordon, served as a nurse and midwife. After earning his MD from the University of Toronto in 1938, he went on to complete his surgical residency at Toronto General Hospital. During the Second World War, he served as a surgeon in casualty clearing stations, which sparked his interest in the effects of injury caused by hypothermia. Once the war was over, Bigelow went to Johns Hopkins University for further studies. He later returned to the Toronto General Hospital and the University of Toronto, all the while examining the physiological effects of hypothermia.

He concluded that cooling patients before surgery would reduce the amount of oxygen the body required, slowing down circulation, finally permitting longer and safer access to the heart. He tested his theory successfully on a dog in 1949. In 1950, the results were presented at an American Surgical Association meeting, and in three years' time, the hypothermia technique was successfully used on a human, making open-heart surgery possible.

His next contribution to cardiac surgery came in the form of the development of the pacemaker. According to the journal of the British Medical Association, in 1949, during experimental surgery, he found he was able to restart a dog's heart by stimulating it at regular intervals with a probe. The following year, he co-developed the first electronic heart pacemaker with Dr Callaghan and electrical engineer John Hopps.

He wrote over 120 papers and two books – *Cold Hearts* and *Mysterious Heparin*. Bigelow was also a surgical teacher at the Toronto General Hospital and the University of Toronto, training cardiac surgeons for over three decades. He also set up the first Division of Cardiac Surgery in Toronto in 1947. One of the most distinguished surgeons from Canada, he received dozens of awards during the course of his career. The International Gairdner Award for Medical Science, the Officer of the Order of Canada, and the F.N.G. Starr Medal – the Canadian Medical Association's highest honour – are just a few of the awards presented to him. He was also the director of the Audubon Society and the Nature Conservancy of Canada.

Fondly known as 'Bill', the pioneering surgeon passed away in 2005.

[8]
RENÉ GERÓNIMO FAVALORO

An Argentine cardiovascular surgeon best remembered for his contributions to coronary bypass surgery, René Gerónimo Favaloro also made immeasurable contributions towards uplifting the quality of healthcare in his country. Favaloro was born in 1923 in La Plata, capital of the province of Buenos Aires. He was of Italian descent and his father worked as a carpenter and his mother as a dressmaker. He completed his secondary education in the famous Colegio Nacional de La Plata and went on to study medicine in the Medical Science Faculty of La Plata University in 1941. He was enamoured by the specialty of surgery and presented his thesis, graduating at the top of his class in 1948 and earning the title of Doctor in Medicine. Favaloro was particularly impressed with his professors Federico Christmann and José Mar'a Mainetti, both masters of surgery.

Hoping to satiate his growing interest in thoracic surgery, he travelled to the city of Buenos Aires once a week to be a part of a postgraduate course on pulmonary and oesophageal surgery. However, due to the political situation of the time, he had to be satisfied with being a country doctor at Jacinto Aráuz, a town in Hucal in the La Pampa Province of Argentina. He used this time rather effectively, indulging in many new things. He began experimenting with preventive medicine and familiarized his patients with basic concepts of hygiene in order to keep diseases at bay. He performed several surgeries and also helped set up the first blood donation centre in the area, which was a major achievement.

Witnessing his interest in cardiovascular surgery, his seniors recommended him for a residency at the Cleveland Clinic in Ohio. However, there were no responses. Eager to learn more, in February 1962, Favaloro arrived unannounced to meet with surgeon George Washington Crile, one of the founders of the Cleveland Clinic. He would say of his experience later: 'I was 38 years old, and I had as a treasure the large experience accumulated in hundreds and hundreds of operations.'

Seeing his enthusiasm, Crile called upon Donald B. Effler, Head of Cardiac Surgery. Favaloro was then accepted as a special trainee, marking the beginning of the most eventful phase of his career. In 1960, using the left internal thoracic artery, a little-known German surgeon Robert Hans Goetz had performed the first successful clinical coronary artery bypass graft surgery in New York. He did not repeat the surgery again even though the operation was a success and the patient lived angina-free for a year before he finally died. Seven years later, in 1967, Favaloro modified the technique and used it on a patient with an occlusion on her right coronary artery. The surgeon conducted a saphenous aortocoronary bypass, which essentially involved using a vein from the patient's leg to reroute the blood flow around the blockage. So far, only mammary veins had been used in the developing procedure. According to the journal of the Texas Heart Institute, Denton Cooley wrote in his tribute to Favaloro: 'Although he was always hesitant to carry the moniker of "father" of coronary artery bypass surgery, he is the surgeon we should credit with introducing coronary bypass surgery into the clinical arena.'

He returned to his home country in 1971 and was determined to create a quality scientific institution dedicated to medical care, training, and research – something on the lines of the Cleveland Clinic. And thus, the Favaloro Foundation was born in 1975 with the help of some supporters. Several courses, meetings, seminars, and conferences would be organized by the foundation to raise the standard of cardiac care in the country. For his work, Favaloro was awarded with several prestigious titles and was also a member of countless medical societies. He was presented with the John Scott Prize in 1979; the creation of the Chair of Cardiovascular Surgery 'Dr René G. Favaloro' by Tel Aviv University, Israel in 1980; the Teacher Prize of Argentinian Medicine in 1986; the Distinguished Alumnus Award of the Cleveland Clinic Foundation in 1987; the René Leriche Prize 1989 by the International Surgery Society; the Gifted Teacher Award by the American College of Cardiology in 1992; the Golden Plate Award of the American Academy of Achievement in 1993; and the Prince Mahidol Award by His Majesty the King of Thailand in 1999.

Favaloro died on 29 July 2000 after committing suicide at the age of 77. Owing to the economic recession and political turmoil in Argentina, the Favaloro Foundation was heavily under debt. Although he asked the government for help to keep things afloat, they did not respond. Finally, fed up of the situation, he shot himself.

On 12 July 2019, on what would have been his 96th birthday, he was honoured through a Google doodle.

[9]

SIR BRIAN BARRATT-BOYES

Sir Brian Barratt-Boyes earned international acclaim as the surgeon who performed New Zealand's first open-heart surgery. He put together a solid team to conduct heart surgeries and pioneered new surgical techniques for the replacement of defective heart valves. He led the way in the development of cardiopulmonary bypass surgery in 1958 in New Zealand and was one of the first surgeons to implant a pacemaker in the human heart before these devices became available commercially in 1961. Owing to his own attempts to quit smoking and a resultant struggle with heart disease, he was all the more empathetic to his patients.

Barratt-Boyes was born in 1924 in Wellington, and attended the Johnsonville Primary School. He later went to Wellington College for secondary schooling. After a year at Victoria University College, he narrowed in on medicine and began his studies at Otago University's Medical School, graduating in 1946. Part of his training as a surgeon was in New Zealand, after which he was off to the Mayo Clinic in Rochester, Minnesota. Once he was back in New Zealand in 1957, he joined the Green Lane Hospital in Auckland, where he was recruited by Sir Douglas Robb, the nation's pioneer of heart surgery and Chancellor of Auckland University. It was the beginning of a long-lasting and rewarding professional relationship.

He turned down dozens of lucrative offers from hospitals and universities in several countries, and remained at Green Lane until 1988, the year of his retirement.

Barratt-Boyes conducted New Zealand's first cardiopulmonary bypass in 1958, making use of an imported Melrose Heart-Lung machine developed at the Postgraduate Medical School, Hammersmith, London. He was a master at overcoming technical issues and demonstrated this quality in 1961, when he became one of the world's first surgeons to implant pacemakers before they were commercially available. These pacemakers were constructed in the workshop of the Auckland University. The next year, he earned the title of being the second heart surgeon in the world to replace a heart valve.

In 1965, a challenging case of a blue baby was handled by him and his team at the hospital. It was hailed as the first successful heart operation in New Zealand and was performed on a three-year-old boy. Barratt-Boyes inserted a portion of tissue into his heart that routed oxygen-charged blood in the right direction instead of going back to the lungs. After this case, he became a champion of similar such paediatric complications involving congenital heart defects. Another notable achievement of the New Zealand surgeon was pioneering what is now a standard procedure of lowering the temperature of babies during heart surgery in 1985.

He was a celebrated figure in New Zealand and his achievements were acknowledged through several prestigious awards. In 1966, he was appointed a Commander of the Order of the British Empire and promoted to Knight Commander of the same order in 1971.

Sir Brian Barratt-Boyes died at the age of 82 in 2006.

[10]
ALBERT STARR

Albert Starr's bold and meticulously timed technique for inserting prosthetic heart valves into patients made him a name to reckon with in heart surgery. It began to be used by surgeons around the world. Starr, along with engineer Miles Lowell Edwards, also invented the first workable prosthesis for the substitution of a cardiac valve. It offered a new lease of life to patients whose lives could be drastically cut short by diseased heart valves. One of his patients from Vancouver survived as many as 50 years with the help of the Starr-Edwards valve. The cardiothoracic surgeon was also instrumental in the invention of the first durable artificial mitral valve in the world and is a co-inventor of the world's first artificial heart valve.

Born in 1926 in New York City, he completed his schooling in a public school in the city, emerging as an exceptional student. He graduated from Columbia University College of Physicians and Surgeons and landed at the Johns Hopkins Hospital for his internship. It was here that he witnessed in action the legendary Alfred Blalock, the man behind the 'blue baby operation'. Blalock's surgery of reconstructing a deformed heart was a leap forward in the treatment of children with congenital heart disease, and Starr got a chance to observe his skills as a surgeon as he conducted the intricate procedure.

Starr entered the US Army Medical Corps in 1952 and was sent off to Korea, where he performed numerous battlefield operations in a mobile army surgical hospital. It turned out to be a profound learning experience for the young surgeon. 'It was a dangerous place, but it was very exciting. I was a battalion surgeon for a few months before I went to a mobile hospital. Those guys were fearless. It was marvelous to see devoted, well-educated men who took the war seriously and were professionals. The experience was eye-opening and had a great effect on me,' he said in an interview.

After the Korea chapter of his life, he resumed training as a general, thoracic, and cardiac surgeon at Presbyterian and Bellevue Hospitals in New York. At just 31 years of age, Starr was recruited to helm an open-heart surgery programme at the University of Oregon's Medical School in Portland, which is now known as Oregon Health Sciences University. This was in the mid-1950s when advancements in cardiopulmonary bypass machines allowed surgeons to open the heart and perform complex procedures in children suffering from deadly congenital heart defects. Dick Sleeter, director of the Crippled Children's Division at the Oregon Medical School, wanted to hire a congenital heart surgeon. Starr stepped in and successfully closed a hole in the inner wall of the heart of a child at University Hospital, making it Oregon's first paediatric open-heart surgery. Inspired as he was by Blalock, he committed himself to congenital heart disease surgery to help these children live a normal life.

Miles Lowell Edwards, a retired engineer, had asked Starr to work with him in testing a mechanical heart. The surgeon, however, convinced him to focus on perfecting a mechanical valve to substitute diseased heart valves. By 1960, the duo had achieved success with an operative and resilient prosthetic valve. Starr then worked on figuring out a surgical procedure to insert the prosthesis efficiently. Later that year, in September, he conducted the first successful mitral valve replacement. The Starr-Edwards prosthetic valve was an innovative development and remained a treatment of choice for over 30 years.

Among his many awards are the Golden Plate Award of the American Academy of Achievement in 1972, the Lasker Award in 2007, and the Scientific Grand Prize of the Lefoulon-Delalande Fondation in 2015.

He remained active in medicine till the age of 90, serving as a scientific advisor to Oregon Heart, involved in the development of a totally artificial heart.

THREE

GAME CHANGERS OF NEUROSURGERY

ONCE UPON A TIME, NEUROSURGERY WAS ONLY about making incisions into the head for pain relief. According to a feature 'Neurosurgery in India' in the *Journal of Postgraduate Medicine*, its history in India is rather interesting and dates back to the mythological era: 'The transplantation of head of an elephant on Ganesha (an Indian Diety), trepanation and removal of intracranial mass by Jivaka (physician to the Lord Buddha) and the neurosurgical accomplishments of Sushruta, the master surgeon, are all documented in the Sushruta Samhita.'

While the specialty has been around for ages, significant developments have only occurred within the last hundred years, making the present an exciting time for neurosurgery. Today, diseases that are treatable through neurosurgery are now being identified, diagnosed, and referred in a timely manner. The advent of several ancillary diagnostic facilities has eased the treatment process, making early neurological intervention highly feasible. The development of minimally invasive technologies, as well as the invention of sophisticatedly crafted surgical tools, has also made a valid contribution to the progress of the specialty.

The fascinating and highly complex nervous system has a very important role to play in our primal survival. It has never been easy to operate upon – one foul move and the patient can lose one of the senses or mobility. However, these masters of the science having honed their skills to perfection, making it seem easy.

[1]
WILDER PENFIELD

If it weren't for Wilder Penfield, modern neurosurgery would have never grown into the sophisticated field it is today. Known for mapping the human brain, Penfield illustrated which parts of it are most strongly linked with various functions such as the five senses, types of body movements, and speech. A neurosurgeon at the University of Montreal, Canada, Penfield was a pioneer in surgery to treat intractable epilepsy. He performed brain surgery to take away the area of the brain causing the uncontrollable seizures typical of the disease. He was sure that just before the seizure, patients experience an 'aura', a kind of indication that the seizure is about to take place. If this aura could be provoked with a mild electric current on the brain, then the source of the seizure activity could be located and that particular bit of tissue could be removed. His fixation with the brain and its mysterious workings led him to research tumours, brain scars, and the several forms of epilepsy. He also explained the phenomenon of déjà vu.

Born in Spokane, Washington, USA, in 1891, Penfield mostly grew up in Hudson, Wisconsin. At the age of 13, his mother suggested he apply for the Rhodes Scholarship. He was successful and attended Merton College, Oxford, where he decided to study medicine, following in the footsteps of his grandfather and estranged father.

Unfortunately, due to an injury he had to leave things midway, but he returned later to complete the course. Penfield completed his medical studies at Johns Hopkins University, receiving his medical degree in 1918. He then worked briefly as a surgical intern at the Peter Bent Brigham Hospital in Boston. He later got the opportunity to assist the brilliant brain surgeon Harvey Cushing.

In 1928, he came to Canada after spending years of training at Oxford, Spain, Germany, and New York. He became the first neurosurgeon in Montreal as he joined the medical faculty of McGill University and also served at the Royal Victoria and Montreal General Hospitals. He wished to establish a neurological institute where surgeons, laboratory researchers, physiologists, and all scientists in the field of neurology could work under one roof. After years of relentless hard work, he was able to set up the Montreal Neurological Institute in 1934.

His technique was often successful, but his experimental surgeries would lead him to new discoveries. One such discovery was the effect of stimulation anywhere on the cerebral cortex could bring forth responses of some kind or the other. He also discovered that only by stimulating the temporal lobes could meaningful, integrated responses be prompted. These included memory, including sound, movement, and colour. If the same areas were stimulated again and again, precisely the same memory would pop up – such as a song, nostalgic imagery, and the like.

Penfield, with this experiment, could prove that there is a physical basis for memory.

According to the *Indian Journal of Psychiatry*, 'his surgical studies yielded reports on brain tumours, the pial circulation, the mechanisms of headache, the localization of motor, sensory and speech functions, and the role of the hippocampus in memory.'

Penfield was the recipient of several awards and honorary degrees. He was also called 'the greatest living Canadian'. He passed away in 1976. His autobiography, *No Man Alone*, which he finished just a few weeks before his death, was published in 1977.

[2]
WALTER EDWARD DANDY

The outstanding Walter Edward Dandy is widely considered as one of the founding fathers of neurosurgery and paediatric neurosurgery. According to the Congress of Neurological Surgeons, he has been credited with several critical discoveries, including the description of the circulation of cerebrospinal fluid in the brain, surgical treatment of hydrocephalus, the description of brain endoscopy, and the first clipping of an intracranial aneurysm. Walter Dandy also researched extensively on abnormalities in the developing human brain. The first clinical description of the Dandy-Walker Syndrome was a result of his collaboration with paediatrician Kenneth Blackfan to understand a congenital brain malformation in which the cerebellar vermis, or the medial part of the brain, is missing. Another major area of research and experimentation for him was the circulation of the cerebral spinal fluid, which surrounds and cushions the brain and spinal cord. He performed numerous pituitary surgeries and also introduced ventriculography to image brain lesions, earning him a nomination for the coveted Nobel Prize.

Dandy was born in 1886 in Sedalia, Missouri. His parents, Rachel Kilpatrick Dandy and engineer John Dandy, were immigrants from Lancashire, England. He graduated as class valedictorian from Summit High School in Sedalia in 1903 and then he was off to the University of Missouri in Columbia, Missouri. After completing his BA in biology in 1907, he pursued a medical degree from Johns Hopkins School of Medicine in Baltimore, Maryland.

At Johns Hopkins, he was asked to study in detail a preserved early stage tow-millimetre human embryo. The results were published in 1910. After that publication, neurosurgeon Harvey Cushing, who was also the founder of the Hunterian Laboratory at Johns Hopkins, hired Dandy as a surgical assistant in his laboratory. Here, he studied the brains of several animals, like cats and dogs, with a focus on the blood supply of the brain and its flow to the pituitary gland. After Dandy graduated from

Johns Hopkins School of Medicine at the age of 24, he started his residency in neurosurgery at Johns Hopkins Hospital under Cushing. The two worked to uncover the forces behind hydrocephalus, the accumulation of cerebral spinal fluid within the brain. However, with differences growing between Cushing and Dandy and the former moving to Harvard, the research was left to the newcomer. He collaborated with Blackfan and their results on the subject were published in two studies in 1913 and 1917.

Dandy was hired as an associate professor of surgery at the Johns Hopkins School of Medicine and assistant visiting surgeon at the hospital in 1921. It was a position he would hold until his retirement despite several lucrative offers from other hospitals of equal standing. In 1931, he rose to the position of clinical professor of neurosurgery at Johns Hopkins.

He developed techniques for the surgical removal of brain tumors and brain aneurisms. With the help of a stellar 'brain team' set up by him, he would perform as many as 1,000 neurosurgeries every year. For malignant tumours, he came up with a new treatment method in 1933, wherein he removed the entire cerebral hemisphere. In 1937, he became the first to perform surgical clipping, also called ligation, of an intracranial aneurysm in the brain. Dandy's procedures were performed by doctors well into the twenty-first century. He was presented with several awards, including the John Scott Award in 1943, for his work in creating ventriculography.

He died in 1946 at the Johns Hopkins Hospital, just before his 60th birthday.

[3]
BALASUBRAMANIAM RAMAMURTHI

A neurosurgeon par excellence, Professor Balasubramaniam Ramamurthi is widely regarded as the father of Indian neurosurgery and made significant efforts for the establishment of the specialty in the country. He was one of the four founding members of the Neurological Society of India and later served as its President. He was also the President of the Association of Surgeons of India. He was born in 1922, at Sirkazi (Shiyali) in the northern part of Tanjore District of Tamil Nadu. His father Captain (Dr) T.S. Balasubramanian was a medical practitioner in Trichinopoly and would travel via bullock cart to see patients. His mother died when Ramamurthi was five; however, he shared a fond relationship with Savithri, his father's second wife.

He studied at the E. R. High School at Trichy and later joined St. Joseph's College for bachelors of Science. He was a gifted student and obtained the highest marks awarded by the University in Mathematics. For his medical studies, he was accepted at the Madras Medical College, graduating in 1943. Throughout his academic career, he won several awards and prizes. At Madras Medical

College, he bagged the Johnstone Medal for securing the first rank. After deciding to specialize in surgery, he joined post-graduate study under Prof. N. S. Narsimha Iyer and earned his MS degree in 1947. Ramamurthi went to Edinburgh in 1947, and in only three months, he qualified for the Fellowship of the Royal College of Surgeons. During his time at Newcastle, he visited other important neurosurgical centres in Europe like Zurich and Stockholm, where he acquainted himself with the stars of neurosurgery of the time such as Krayenbuhl, Olivecrona, Edward Busch, Gosta V. Norlen and Lars Leksell. In 1950, he spent six months at the respected Montreal Neurological Institute in Montreal, Canada.

Finally, in October 1950, Ramamurthi headed back home and joined as an assistant surgeon at the Madras Medical College. He came back to his alma mater to promote the specialty, which was still in its infancy in the country. After persistent efforts, four beds in the general surgery ward were expanded to create an independent ward and operation theatre for neurosurgery. It would eventually take the form of the Madras Neurological Institute. In 1960, Ramamurthi agreed to operate upon Andhra Pradesh Governor General Shrinagesh, who was suffering from Parkinson's disease. Shrinagesh had already been operated upon on one side. Now it was the other side of the brain that required surgery. Ramamurthi requested for some equipment and was provided approval by Pandit Jawaharlal Nehru to invite Mr Lawrence

Walsh along with purchasing all the required equipment under the Commonwealth Aids Scheme. This marked the beginning of the stereotaxy unit, which would gain international recognition in the years to follow.

He established other centres for the advancement of neurosurgery in India, such as the National Brain Research Centre in Manesar, Haryana, and the Dr Achanta Lakshipathi Neurological Centre, to which he devoted the final 25 years of his life. He also played important roles in establishing the Middle East Neurosurgical Society, the Asian Australasian Association of Neurosurgeons, and the South Asian Association of Neurosurgeons. He gathered an exhaustive number of awards, including the Padma Shri in 1972 and the Padma Bhushan and 1977, India's fourth- and third-highest civilian honours respectively. He was the honorary President of the World Federation of Neurosurgical Societies and an honorary member of the Australian Society of Neurosurgeons; Society of Neurological Surgeons, USA; American Academy of Neurosurgeons; Japanese Neurosurgical Society; Scandinavian Neurosurgical Society; and the Congress of Neurological Surgeons. He was also presented with the John Bruce Gold Medal of the Royal College of Surgeons of Edinburgh.

He passed away in 2003 at the age of 81.

[4]
M. GAZI YAŞARGIL

Known as the father of microneurosurgery, M. Gazi Yaşargil earned international fame and recognition for his treatment of epilepsy and brain tumours using his own instruments. He redefined neurosurgery and made previously inoperable conditions treatable with a team of skilled surgeons. During the course of his career, he has performed more than 7,500 impressive intracranial surgeries successfully.

Born in 1925 in Lice, a village in eastern Turkey, Yaşargil and his family moved to Ankara when he was very young as his parents wanted to provide their children access to its excellent educational institutions. Yaşargil attended Ankara public schools, graduating in 1943. He became familiar with medicine and neurology as one of his father's friends was a neurologist. In 1944, he entered medical school at Frederick Schiller University in Jena, Germany. Following the disruption of classes in 1945 because of the Second World War, he transferred to medical school at Basel, Switzerland, earning his medical degree in 1950.

Yaşargil met Professor Hugo Krayenbühl, Head of Neurosurgery at the University of Zurich, and was immediately in awe of him and the way he passionately spoke of the finer details of the nervous system. He joined Krayenbühl in neurological surgery in 1953. However, he was quite dissatisfied with the available macrosurgical techniques and felt that there had to be another way. He also grew very interested in new technology such as angiography and thought it could have useful applications in neurosurgery. Using the technique of microsurgery allowed access and visibility to lesions by means of a dissecting microscope; they appeared magnified. The study of the surgery of such minute structures was being conducted in the United States, and the young Turkish doctor wanted to be a part of it. Upon Krayenbühl's request, an arrangement was made with the Microvascular Laboratory at the University of Vermont in Burlington. Yaşargil joined the research staff in 1965 and worked there for about a year and a half. It paved a new way for him and for neurosurgery.

According to the Congress of Neurological Surgeons, he conceived the idea of using the superficial temporal artery as a direct connection into a middle cerebral branch that did not involve the removal of a segment of the superficial temporal artery, and hence did not require a double suture line. The superficial temporal vessel was simply sectioned far enough out to allow it to be sutured to the middle cerebral branch by a single end-to-side anastomosis. This technique provided a greatly improved patency rate, and the results were reported in 1967.

His extensive study and research of the subarachnoid spaces is well revered by the neurosurgery fraternity. He showed that several – if not most – intracranial operations can be done in the subarachnoid space with an intact pia and arachnoid to achieve low mortality and morbidity rates.

According to the journal *Neurosurgery*, 'To enable the advancement of microsurgical techniques, Yaşargil created innovative instrumentation, such as the floating microscope, the self-retaining adjustable retractor, microsurgical instruments, and ergonomic aneurysm clips and appliers. His genius in developing microsurgical techniques for use in cerebrovascular neurosurgery has transformed the outcomes of patients with conditions that were previously inoperable.'

He has published more than 300 papers as well as some textbooks. Needless to say, he has earned several awards and accolades, the most noteworthy being Neurosurgery's Man of the Century 1950–1999 at the Congress of Neurological Surgeons Annual Meeting in 1999.

Yaşargil spent most of his career at the University of Zurich, which he joined in 1953 as resident, ultimately rising to the position of chief resident and then professor and chairman of the department of neurosurgery, University of Zurich and the Zurich University Hospital. He retired after 40 years in 1993 but continues to be active, accepting a position as a professor of neurosurgery at the University of Arkansas's College of Medicine. He also remains involved in research.

[5]
KARIN MURASZKO

The extraordinary paediatric neurosurgeon who has herself battled the lifelong spinal cord abnormality of spina bifida, Karin Muraszko was the first woman to be accepted as a neurosurgery resident at Columbia University. She was also the first neurosurgery resident at Columbia Presbyterian Medical Center with a physical disability. In 2005, when she was appointed Chair of Neurosurgery at the University of Michigan, she became the first woman in the United States to hold such a position. She was also the first woman appointed as a Director of the American Board of Neurological Surgeons. Muraszko specializes in paediatric neurosurgery, including paediatric brain and central nervous system tumours, and paediatric spine surgery. She has researched extensively on experimental therapies for paediatric brain tumours, management of Chiari malformations, and other congenital abnormalities of the spine and brain. She has also been dedicated to the treatment of children with complex craniofacial anomalies.

Born in 1955 in Jersey City, New Jersey, Muraszko graduated from Yale University with a double major in history and biology in 1977. She then joined the Columbia College of Physicians and Surgeons, passing out in 1981. She also completed her residency training in neurological surgery, as well as fellowships in paediatric neurosurgery, at the Neurological Institute of New York in the New York-Presbyterian/Columbia University Medical Center. After completing her training in 1988, she immersed herself in research working as a Senior Staff Fellow at the National Institutes of Health in the Surgical Neurology Branch for two years.

Since 1990, Muraszko has been associated with the University of Michigan, becoming Chief of the Pediatric Neurosurgery Service in 1995. Finally, in 2005, she rose to the position of the chair of the department of neurosurgery. She is a member of the American Association of Neurological Surgeons and the Congress of Neurological Surgeons. She is also involved in various paediatric professional associations and is the director of the Pediatric Brain Tumor Clinic at the University of Michigan Comprehensive Cancer Center. Muraszko is the co-founder of Project Shunt, which works to provide care to destitute children in Guatemala. She is an active member of the Physician's Advisory Committee of the Spina Bifida Association and the March of Dimes. She also works as a professor in the department of neurosurgery with joint appointments in plastic surgery and paediatrics.

She credits her success to her parents who didn't abandon her due to her condition and saw her as capable, instead of handicapped. However, in the male-dominated profession she chose for herself, gender inequalities emerged as a bigger challenge in comparison to her physical disability. In a CNN interview, Muraszko said, 'People often ask me which has been harder – being a woman neurosurgeon or having a disability as a surgeon. Being a woman was more difficult.'

In 2015, Muraszko began losing function in her legs, requiring another surgery. She is still working, though not actively as a surgeon since she is now in a wheelchair. However, her tenacity and spirit remain fiercely alive.

She lives in Ann Arbor in Michigan with her husband and two children.

[6]
HIROTARO NARABAYASHI

The founder of stereotactic neurosurgery in Japan, Hirotaro Narabayashi was among of the first few pioneers of this field in the world. He constructed his first stereotactic apparatus in 1949, which he used to perform his first pallidotomy in 1951. Since Japan was just recovering from war, he was unacquainted with similar work being done outside his country. He set up his own private neurological clinic in Tokyo in 1957, which became an international hub for stereotaxy and attracted neurosurgeons and patients from round the world for over 40 years.

Narabayashi was born in Kobe, Japan in 1922, spending his childhood in Nagasaki. After graduating from the Graduate School of Medicine, University of

Tokyo, after World War II, he joined Professor Y. Uchimura's department of psychiatry (neurosurgery was clubbed with psychiatry in Japan in those days). Ogawa showed him some drawings of Horsley and Clarke's stereotaxic apparatus that were being used in animal experiments. Upon hearing his suggestion to use the same on humans, Narabayashi sprung to action, eager to work on it. However, after the post-war chaos, Tokyo had been ravaged by bombardment. After a lot of hunting and legwork, he found a small factory that was ready to help him, and that's how his first stereotactic instrument was manufactured in 1949 and reported in Kyoto in 1950. This model was not used on humans; revised models that followed in the coming few years were. Though Earnest Spiegel and Henry Wycis reported the first human stereotactic procedure in 1947, Japan was occupied by America and communication with other countries was largely cut off, with doctors having no access to foreign journals. Working independently, he developed stereotaxy in post-war Japan.

Narabayashi first applied his indigenous instrument for a pallidotomy in an athetoid child in 1951. In 1952, the first pallidotomy was performed by him on Parkinson's disease and it was a great success, with the patient's tremors and rigidity almost vanishing. It was the third operation on this patient, with the previous ones conducted by other surgeons not yielding significant results. Seeing the amazing results, Narabayashi devoted the rest of his career to the development and applications of stereotaxy.

It is to Narabayashi's credit that neurosurgery departments were established in the university hospitals steadily, and stereotactic surgery was being hailed as a new idea and method. He stood at the epicentre of this process and established a private clinic in 1957, focusing exclusively on stereotaxic neurosurgery, which became world-renowned for both research and treatment. Meanwhile, he also served as associate professor of psychiatry and later as full professor of neurology at Juntendo University in Tokyo. He travelled far and wide to several countries to talk about his methods and instruments and participated in countless conferences. He performed a staggering 4,000 stereotactic procedures in his life.

In 1989, he was presented with the Spiegel and Wycis Medal for his work towards the development of Stereotactic and Functional Surgery. He was also elected Honorary Member of several foreign medical societies such as the American and French Societies of Neurology.

Unfortunately, he suffered a left retinal haemorrhage in April 2000, losing most of his central vision, and could not continue performing surgeries. The same year, his wife died. Unable to bear this loss, he passed five months after her demise in 2001.

[7]

BASANT KUMAR MISRA

The first in South Asia to perform Gamma Knife radiosurgery and the first in the world to perform computer-guided aneurysm surgery, Basant Kumar Misra has a lot of firsts to his credit. He was the first Indian to conduct an 'awake' craniotomy as well as laparoscopic spine surgery. His other areas of proficiency in neurosurgical patient care include acoustic neuroma surgery, vascular neurosurgery, skull base surgery, pituitary surgery, minimally invasive neurosurgery, and complex brain and spine disorders.

He was born in 1953 in Bhubaneshwar, Odisha, to Basanti Misra and Professor Baidyanath Misra, who was a renowned economist and served as the Vice Chancellor of Orissa University of Agriculture and Technology and the Deputy Chairman of State Planning Board, Orissa. After completing his early education in Bhubaneshwar, he pursued MBBS from V. S. S. Medical College, Sambalpur University in Burla, Odisha and passed out in 1975. He was presented with the award of Best Graduate of the university and four gold medals. Thereafter, he completed his masters in general surgery at Safdarjang Hospital, New Delhi in 1980 and Master of Chirurgie (MCh) in neurosurgery at the All India Institute of Medical Sciences, New Delhi, in 1983. He received the Commonwealth Medical Scholarship to the University of Edinburgh, United Kingdom, and is a proud recipient of the Pfizer Post Graduate Medical Award.

While he began his career as a research officer at the Indian Council of Medical Research, he is currently fulfilling many roles at Hinduja Hospitals, Mumbai, India. He is the Chairman and Chief of Surgery, and Head of the neurosurgery department and has treated several eminent personalities, including Bollywood celebrities like Hrithik Roshan and Salman Khan.

An international leader held in high esteem, he has been actively involved in a number of professional societies. He has served as the President of the Neurological Society India, Skull Base Surgery Society of India, and the Cerebrovascular Society of India. He was the elected the second Vice President of the World Federation of Neurosurgical Societies. He was the first Indian to be elected President of Asian Australasian Society of Neurological Surgeons and President of International Conference of Cerebrovascular Societies. He was the first Asian to be President of the World Federation of Skull Base Societies. Few others in the profession have held so many leading positions. Following in the footsteps of the late Balasubramaniam Ramamurthi, he became only the second Indian member of the American Academy of Neurological Surgery. Being listed as 'One of the World's Top 16 Neurosurgeons That Matter' by *Jo Lee Magazine*, New York, in 2015, was another feather in his cap. Misra has also been presented with the B. C. Roy Award, the highest medical honour in India.

Misra works and lives in Mumbai with his wife. They have two sons who work and live abroad.

[8]
HENRY MARSH

Henry Marsh, a celebrated British neurosurgeon who has spent four decades operating on the brain, worked tirelessly to promote neurosurgery in communities in Ukraine and Nepal. Henry Marsh also pioneered the use of 'awake' brain surgery along with cortical mapping in such surgery. He can boast of being the neurosurgeon to perform the highest number of these procedures in the UK and one of the highest in Europe. His impressive body of work in Ukraine, spanning over two decades, was the subject of the documentary film *The English Surgeon*, which went on to win an Emmy in 2010.

Born in 1950 in Oxford, UK, Marsh attended the Dragon School in Oxford and the Westminster School in London. Interestingly, medicine wasn't the first priority on his mind as he studied politics, philosophy, and economics at University College, Oxford University in 1969, where he achieved first class honours. He then veered towards medicine, graduating with honours in medicine from the Royal Free Medical School. He had just qualified as a junior doctor when his three-month-old son was diagnosed with a brain tumour. He was operated on a week later and he recovered.

Watching William survive the complicated removal of his brain tumour, Marsh made the decision to specialize in neurosurgery. Going through the nerve-wracking experience in the early stage of his medical career proved to be a blessing in disguise, and helped him empathize better with the families of his patients.

He became a fellow of the Royal College of Surgeons in 1984 and began serving as a consultant neurosurgeon at the Atkinson Morley Wing at St George's Hospital, where he would spend most of his career. While he retired from full-time surgical work at St George's in 2015, he continued his association with hospitals in Ukraine and Nepal. He has actively been collaborating with neurosurgeons in Ukraine, most of all with his protégé Igor Kurilets, as association that began in 1992. He is also clinical professor of neurosurgery at the University of Washington in Seattle, USA, and Honorary Consultant Neurosurgeon to the Royal Marsden Hospital in London and the University of Wales in Cardiff. He was also involved with the National Health Service, retiring in 2019.

Belonging to a literary family, writing came naturally to him – and it wasn't just research papers. Marsh has written two highly acclaimed memoirs. Published in 2014, *Do No Harm: Stories of Life, Death and Brain Surgery* became an international bestseller. In 2017, another memoir, *Admissions: Life as a Brain Surgeon*, was released. Over the course of his career spanning over

40 years, Marsh has earned several awards and honours. He was appointed Commander of the Order of the British Empire in 2010. The same year, he presented the Leslie Oliver Oration at the Queen's Hospital.

He lives with his second wife, social anthropologist and author Kate Fox, dividing their time between their homes in Oxford and south London.

[9]
JOHN R. ADLER

A surgeon-entrepreneur who holds nine patents, John R. Adler is the inventor of the CyberKnife, a precision tool used for invasive surgeries that has revolutionized neurosurgery in recent times. With the clever use of imaging, it can actually get rid of tumours and lesions with minimal surgical intervention. Apart from CyberKnife, he has published more than 180 peer-reviewed chapters and articles, becoming one of the most published neurosurgeons in the world.

Born in Yonkers, New York, in 1954, Adler graduated from Harvard College in 1976 and from Harvard Medical School in 1980. A neurosurgical residency at Massachusetts General Hospital and Brigham and Women's Hospital followed. He was very keen on the practical implications of radiosurgery in his specialty and completed a radiosurgery fellowship at the Karolinska Institute in Sweden in 1985, where he worked closely with Lars Leksell, which changed the shape of his career. Leksell had invented the Gamma Knife for targeted radiation to brain tumours. While Adler was impressed, he also saw room for improvement. Since the Gamma Knife depended on a physical cage to coordinate the position of the subject's head with the device supplying the radiation, Adler thought that medical images to guide the beam would do a far better job.

Back in America in 1987, he joined the faculty of Stanford University School of Medicine as an assistant professor in the department of neurosurgery. He began collaborating with faculty in the engineering school to build a prototype of the CyberKnife. He was bitten by the entrepreneurial bug, and by 1987, was propositioning venture capitalists. They rejected his idea and he took it upon himself to raise $800,000 from other neurosurgeons, friends, and family, and started his own company, Accuray, in 1990 to produce the CyberKnife. He also remained on the Stanford faculty.

Owing to his training and experience in radiosurgery, he was also appointed assistant professor in radiation oncology in 1992, promoted to associate professor in the neurosurgery and radiation oncology departments in 1993, and full professor in both departments in 1998. He was named the Dorothy and Thye King Chan Professor in neurosurgery in 2007, eventually being appointed an emeritus professor.

He continues to work in important positions in

several companies that manufacture innovative surgical tools and systems, and has also been associated with various professional societies and institutions. Adler has received several awards such as the Inaugural Ideals of Entrepreneurship Award, Emerging Entrepreneurs in Biomedical Technology, Biodesign Group by Stanford University in 2005; Outstanding Achievement in Medicine by the Santa Clara Valley Medical Association in 2007; Cushing Award for Excellence and Innovation in Neurosurgery by the American Association for Neurological Surgery in 2018; and more.

[10]
ALIM-LOUIS BENABID

While routinely performing lesioning of the thalamus in the brains of patients suffering from severe Parkinson's disease, Alim-Louis Benabid made a revolutionary discovery: he realized that deep brain stimulation could be effective for the treatment of the disease. L-dopa (levodopa), the preferred mode of treatment for the disease during the 1980s, came with its own set of side effects. He achieved lesioning by placing an electrode at the preferred site to burn the brain tissue, experimenting with various frequencies. He tried from very low, starting from 1Hz before going up to 100 Hz. He noticed that at 100 Hz, the tremors were suppressed, and then, Benabid had the final solution.

Born in 1942 in La Tronche, near Grenoble, France, Benabid spent his childhood in Sétif in Algeria. His mother was a French nurse and his father an Algerian doctor. By the time he was old enough to attend secondary school, they were back in Grenoble. Benabid earned his medical degree in 1970 and PhD in physics in 1978. Following a post-doctoral fellowship in the laboratory of pre-clinical neuropharmacology at the Salk Institute in 1979, he was hired as a professor of neurosurgery and experimental medicine at Grenoble University. He remained in the post till 1983, and then taught neurosurgery and biophysics. In 1988, he served as the director of the research laboratory INSERM unit 318 (pre-clinical neurosciences) for almost 19 years. He was also appointed as the head of the neurosurgery department at the University Hospital of Grenoble and professor of biophysics at Joseph Fourier University from 1989 to 2007. For nine years, he was also the coordinator of the Claudio Munari Center for Surgery of Epilepsy and Movement Disorders at Hospital Ni Guardia in Milan, Italy and the staff consultant at the Cleveland Clinic Foundation, Ohio from 2000–2003.

The technological innovation of electrodes into the brain was hailed as a revolutionary discovery by the international scientific community. His team, under his guidance, fashioned a technique that could implant electrodes directly into the brains of patients with Parkinson's to supply high-frequency electrical stimulation and get rid of the motor symptoms associated with the disease, such as tremors. This approach was quite safe, with a low morbidity rate, and could also reduce dependency on drugs.

After the success of deep brain stimulation, Benabid focused on stimulating the subthalamic nucleus in the brain, with animal studies showing promising results for the treatment of Parkinson's disease. His trials proved the results shown in animal studies and deep brain stimulation entered its advanced state.

Benabid has 523 scientific papers and 3 honorary degrees under his belt, and has given 18 honorary lectures. He has been the proud recipient of a whopping 23 medals and coveted prizes including the Dr Pierre Pollak Robert A. Pritzker Prize for Leadership in Parkinson's Research in 2013 and the Lasker Award in 2014. Some of the other noteworthy awards presented to him include the James Parkinson Award, Victor Horsley Award, American Academy of Neurology's Movement Disorders Research Award ,and the European Inventor Award for the research category.

Though he retired in 2007, he is currently overseeing a building project of a new biomedical research centre funded by the French national government with a €3 million grant from the Edmond Safra Foundation.

[illegible]

[illegible]

[illegible]

Though he retired in 1997, he [illegible]

FOUR

STALWARTS OF GASTRO SURGERY

WHETHER IT'S GUT INSTINCT OR A GUT FEELING or butterflies in the stomach, our digestive system has often been connected to the mind and the well-being of our entire body. And it is not without reason. The gut–brain axis governs how various emotions affect the body's ability to process food. The digestive system is indeed a complex one that runs our everyday lives. Since it encompasses a large number of organs like the liver, stomach, intestines, pancreas, gall bladder and more, gastrointestinal surgery is divided into various subspecialties that have all come into their own in the past century.

With significant contributions and advancements in surgical techniques, open surgeries of the gastrointestinal system have become less common. Improvements in anaesthesia and critical care, along with diagnostic radiology, gastroenterology and bioengineering have also shaped modern gastro surgery. What we know today about microbiology and pharmacology due to the efforts of research teams all over the world has also helped manage these conditions better. According to the journal *Surgery*, 'A poignant example is the virtual disappearance of elective surgery for peptic ulcer because of the discovery of powerful acid-suppressing pharmaceutical agents as well as recognition of the etiological significance of Helicobacter pylori eradication.' Of course, pioneers in the field have played a pivotal role in making gastro surgery a highly organized and structured specialty with several subspecialties that are thriving.

[1]
ERICH MÜHE

The German surgeon was the first to perform cholecystectomy or gall bladder removal applying the newly developed technology of laparoscopy in 1985. For the procedure, Erich Mühe designed his own surgical laparoscope in 1984 which he named the 'Galloscope'. The surgery was a success and the surgeon was dumbfounded at the fast rate of recovery of his patient. After conducting 94 such surgeries with positive results, he published his work in 1986 at the Congress of the German Society of Surgery. However, he was met with ridicule when he discussed the revolutionary new approach. Today, he is regarded as a surgeon who was ahead of his time and had the foresight to use the new technology for gall bladder removal surgery.

Born in 1938, Mühe obtained his medical degree in 1966. His surgical training took place at the University of Erlangen–Nuremberg, which he completed in 1973. He then moved to Böblingen and began working as head of the surgical clinic in the Böblingen county hospital in 1982.

According to the *Journal of Laparoscopic and Robotic Surgeons*, he later modified his technique and operated through a trocar sleeve. It led to the development of an 'open laparoscope' with a circular light. His concept, however, was ignored. In the middle of the 1980s, the surgical community was still not prepared for the era of 'minimally invasive therapy'. Nonetheless, he persisted and gave two additional lectures on his technique in 1986 and 1987 and talked about minimized post-operative pain, shorter hospital stays, miniscule incisions and a faster return to the workplace. However, he was met with closed minds and the same unwelcoming response.

The abdominal system with its complicated anatomical structure was still not considered compatible with minimally invasive surgery that had begun to gain popularity in several other specialties of surgery. Adding to the resistance were the advanced level of high-quality drugs coupled with advances in anaesthesia that were all conducive to surgeons wanting to indulge in major and invasive gastro surgeries. It was only in 1992, that Mühe received official honours for pioneering work in endoscopic surgery at the Congress of the German Surgical Society. By then his surgery was already being practiced in several parts of Europe and North America.

Today, his method is the gold standard in the treatment. With just four small incisions and barely any sutures, the patient can go home just a couple of hours after the surgery. Laparoscopic cholecystectomy has even been found to be an efficient treatment for the early stages of gall bladder cancer.

Mühe passed away in 2005, after a carer spent radically changing the approach to cholecystectomy.

[2]
PIER CRISTOFORO GIULIANOTTI

When artificial intelligence meets human capabilities, the results can often be astounding. Pier Cristoforo Giulianotti pioneered the use of then new robotic technology to perform complex gastro surgical procedures such as formal hepatic resection and pancreaticoduodenectomy in 2000. To his credit is also the establishment of one of the biggest and most impressive programmes in the world for robotic surgery – the Special School ACOI of Robotic Surgery. He was honoured with the highly esteemed Lloyd M. Nyhus Endowed Chair in Surgery at the University of Illinois at Chicago in 2007 and has since been appointed to the position of chief of the division of general, minimally invasive and robotic surgery.

Born in 1953 in Filattiera, Tuscany, Giulianotti spent his student years in Italy. He obtained his MD degree from La Scuola Normale of Pisa University in Italy. Apart from a formal general surgery residency, he also completed two more residencies in digestive and vascular surgery. In the mid-1980s he acquainted himself with laparoscopic surgery techniques and established himself as an expert in the same. In 1998, he was appointed as the director of general and minimally invasive surgery at Misericordia Hospital in Grosseto, Tuscany. He also joined the University of Sienna as a professor of surgery the same year. He was fascinated with the newly developing robotic-assisted surgery technology and was eager to apply them in the procedures he was undertaking. In the year 2000 he conducted two robotic-assisted surgeries – robotic total gastrectomy and robotic donor nephrectomy for living donor kidney transplant – becoming the first surgeon to do so in the world. His forays continued and the next year he performed several other surgeries using the technology. These included robotic liver resection, robotic spleen-preserving distal pancreatectomy, robotic Whipple with biliary and digestive reconstruction, robotic ilio-femoral bypass and robotic splenic artery aneurysm repair. Again, he was the first in the world to conduct these surgeries using robotic assistance. At the Misericordia Hospital he was promoted to the position of head of the department of general surgery in 2003.

By this time, other countries had started inviting him to conduct and demonstrate such surgeries. He left Italy in 2007 to join as the vice-head, department of surgery, and the chief, division of general, minimally invasive and robotic surgery, department of surgery at the University of Illinois at Chicago, USA. Another one of his appointments was professor of surgery at the university.

He has published more than 250 papers in scientific journals on various topics including pancreatic, vascular, digestive and robotic surgery. For his contribution as a surgeon and educator, Giulianotti has been the recipient of various awards and honours. He has been elected member of various professional societies such as the International Advisory Board (IAB) for the Japan Robotic Surgery Society (J-ROBO) and the International Advisory Board of the Minimal Access Surgery Training Centre (MASTC), Pamela Youde Nethersole Eastern Hospital in Hong Kong. In 2009 he was listed by Fast Company Magazine as one of the '100 Most Creative People in Business'. In 2013, he earned the Faculty of the Year Award by University of Illinois Hospital and Health Sciences System, College of Medicine.

He continues to work at the University of Illinois in Chicago and has trained countless budding surgeons in the art of robot-assisted surgery.

[3]
EDWARD MASON

Fondly remembered as the 'Father of obesity surgery', Edward Mason played a pivotal role in the development of gastric restrictive surgery to help morbidly obese patients. He was the first to perform gastric bypass in 1966 and also invented the first vertical banded gastroplasty (also known as stomach stapling) in 1980. Mason was of the opinion that obesity was an epidemic that needed to be controlled on a priority basis, as it not only affects the quality of life but also exposes one to sundry ailments such as heart disease, hypertension, diabetes, arthritis, cancer, high cholesterol and strokes.

Mason was born in Boise, Idaho, in 1920 to Edward Files Mason, who was a professor of photojournalism at the University of Iowa and Dora Eaton Mason, who was a teacher and talented sculptress. After graduation from City High in Iowa in 1939, he opted for medical studies and obtained his MD at the University of Iowa in 1945. He briefly served in the navy during the Second World War. Once his service in the war was over, he headed to Minnesota to train under Owen Wangensteen at the University of Minnesota. He particularly studied the surgical treatment of the duodenal ulcer in detail. In 1953, he earned his PhD in surgery and returned to Iowa to join the surgery department at the University of Iowa. In 1981–82 he served as acting head of the department of surgery at the university. Iowa is where he would remain and would ultimately become emeritus professor in 1991.

He collaborated with surgeon Chikashi Ito from Sapporo, Japan, in 1965. The duo conducted a few experiments to figure out how gastric bypass could be used as an effective treatment for peptic ulcer disease. While they concluded that the ulcers were not going anywhere with gastric bypass, there was a pleasant side effect to be observed. They realized that the obese patients were losing weight after the gastric bypass surgery. The roots of bariatric or obesity surgery were sown. Mason was greatly helped by Ito in the process and for this reason, Ito is often referred to as a co-founder of bariatric surgery.

Today the gastric bypass, vertical banded gastroplasty and various permutations and combinations of Mason's surgeries form the cornerstones of the subspecialty of bariatric surgery. They are used all over the world for morbidly obese patients and the treatment of type 2 diabetes and other such metabolic co-morbidities.

Mason was the founder of the American Society for Metabolic and Bariatric Surgery, established in 1983. During the course of his long and eventful career, he worked on more than 200 papers and book chapters and published five books. His last book, an autobiographical account, *A Fat Chance* was published on his 100th birthday.

He passed away in December 2020 at the age of 100.

[4]
ALLEN WHIPPLE

This Iranian-born American surgeon is well known for the pancreatic cancer operation (pancreaticoduodenectomy) or the Whipple procedure, which is named after him. He was the first to perform the operation in 1935. The Whipple's Triad, a set of three criteria that indicate a patient's symptoms arise from hypoglycemia, is also named after him.

Born in 1881 in Urmia, West Azerbaijan, Iran to missionary parents Williaam Levi Whipple and Mary Louise Whipple, Whipple graduated from Princeton

University in 1904. He then graduated from medical school at Columbia's College of Physicians and Surgeons, receiving his MD in 1908. He began his practice in New York in 1910, and in 1921 was appointed as a professor of surgery of the New York-Presbyterian/Columbia Medical Center, New York. He would eventually rise to the rank of surgeon-in-chief and would remain here till 1946.

In 1935 he initiated work on the resection of the pancreas or pancreaticoduodenectomy and emerged successful. The procedure entailed the surgical removal of the wide part of the pancreas, located right next to the first part of the small intestine or duodenum. The procedure also required removing the duodenum, a part of the common bile duct and gallbladder. In some cases a part of the stomach was also required to be removed. The parts of the intestine, bile duct and pancreas that were left behind would finally be reconnected to restore normal digestive function. It emerged as a successful treatment for cancer of the pancreas. In 1940, Whipple simplified and streamlined the procedure.

According to the journal *Digestive Surgery,* 'Many of the great names in surgery in America, continental Europe and the United Kingdom have been associated with the solution of these problems, but towering above them must be Allen Oldfather Whipple, together with his colleagues, at the Columbia-Presbyterian Medical Center, New York. Whipple not only pioneered the radical surgery of pancreatic cancer but clearly characterized the clinical syndrome produced by insulinoma of the pancreas.'

Though he only conducted 37 of these surgeries during his career and his original technique has undergone various modifications, the procedure is still relevant in today's times. He retired in 1946, but continued to teach, write and indulge in research. He also accepted a position on the faculty of the American University of Bierut where he was also a trustee. He supervised the establishment of a new medical centre in Shiraz.

He passed away in 1963 at the age of 81 in New Jersey.

[5]
NATESAN RANGABASHYAM

A Padma Bhushan awardee, Natesan Rangabashyam was a pioneer in surgical gastroenterology who made several contributions towards establishing the specialty and promoting it in India. He was the man behind setting up the first MCh course in surgical gastroenterology in the country in 1984 at the Madras Medical College. He was also a pioneer in proctology, and also set up the first enterostomal therapy diploma to train nursing professionals in the country. Rangabashyam was an honorary surgeon to the president of India as well.

Born in 1936, in Chennai (then Madras), Rangabashyam's father was a general practitioner.

Though he didn't want to follow in his father's footsteps and aspired to be a pilot, Rangabashyam eventually had a change of heart and enrolled at Loyola College in Madras to study natural sciences. After studying medicine at Madras Medical College, he obtained his MBBS in 1957 and was off to the UK. At Edinburgh he joined the primary course at the Royal College of Surgeons there. He served at the Royal Alexandra Hospital in Rhyl, Wales, as a medical officer. Here, he trained in surgical gastroenterology with Ivor Lewis and Owen Daniels, gaining his FRCS Edinburgh in 1963. He gained exposure in a few hospitals in Edinburgh and London thereafter.

Eager to make a difference in his country, he was back in India in 1964, where he was appointed as an honorary surgeon and clinical professor of surgery at Thanjavur Medical College and Hospital in Thanjavur, Tamil Nadu. He set up a gastrointestinal clinic and also began the practice of selective vagotomy procedures. He performed his first hepatic resection here. He joined the Stanley Medical College and Hospital in Chennai in 1969 as a consultant surgeon. Thereafter, in 1975 he was appointed head of the department of surgical gastroenterology and honorary clinical professor of surgery at the Madras Medical College and Government General Hospital.

He made valuable contributions in the treatment of gastrointestinal cancers, colitis, portal hypertension and bowel disease and has written extensively on them, contributing to chapters in textbooks. He also played a major part in organizing the FRCS Edinburgh Examination to be arranged in India and he was successful in 1995.

He has been associated with the Association of Surgeons of India and the Indian Society of Gastroenterology and has also served as their president. A fellow of the International College of Surgeons, the International Academy of Proctology as well as the American College of Surgeons, Rangabashyam is also a member of the Academy of Medicine, Singapore. He won several awards and felicitations and proudly accepted the B.C. Roy Award twice in his career, which is the highest Indian award in medicine.

At the age of 79, Rangabashyam passed away in his sleep, in 2013.

[6]
CHARLES MCBURNEY

The year was 1891 and Charles McBurney had just published a treatise on appendicitis. He had very accurately described the precise location on the abdomen at which the patient experienced the most pain when suffering from acute appendicitis. Today the point is known as 'McBurney's point.' A lot has changed in the management of appendicitis since 1891 and one would think that newer diagnostic technologies would have rendered McBurney's point useless. However, according to the *Journal of Emergency Medicine*, 'Despite these advances, tenderness to palpation over McBurney's point remains a key finding on abdominal examination in the assessment of patients with abdominal pain.' A few years later he also described the muscle-splitting incision he had used in a surgery for the removal of the appendix. That came to be known as McBurney's incision.

Born in 1845 in Roxbury in Boston, Massachusetts, he completed his schooling at the Roxbury Latin School followed by a private school in Boston. He enrolled at Harvard University in 1862 for the Bachelor of Arts course, and afterwards the Master of Arts course. The College of Physicians and Surgeons of New York was his next stop where he received his doctorate in medicine in 1870. When his 18-month residency at Bellevue Hospital was complete, he was off to Europe where he explored various major medical centres. Once back in New York, he started his practice in 1873 and was also appointed as a demonstrator in anatomy at the College of Physicians and Surgeons of New York. He went from strength to strength, eventually earning the title of professor of surgery in 1889 at the age of 44. However, due to his demanding practice, he stepped down from the position a few years later. In 1888 at the Roosevelt Hospital he was appointed as surgeon-in-chief. It was an exhausting role with over 1200 surgeries taking place every year.

McBurney was meticulous about his surgical practices

and was among the early promoters of the use of rubber gloves in the field. He followed antiseptic techniques religiously as he was of the opinion that surgeries on the abdominal cavity could become much safer with their use. He was the first surgeon to elaborate on the point rather eloquently that early surgery for appendicitis was practical and waiting for too long could prove fatal. Though it was British surgeon Lawson Tait who was the first to remove an extremely inflamed appendix, McBurney set up the rules and strategies for the clinical diagnosis and surgical treatment for the now commonplace procedure of appendectomy. His guidelines are still relevant today.

A member of various societies, McBurney was presented with an honorary fellowship in surgical organizations throughout Europe and America. He retired in 1905.

He died in 1913, at the age of 68.

[7] MORIO KASAI

Though technically a paediatric surgeon, Morio Kasai made a significant contribution to the gastro surgery specialty. Regarded as a 'small giant' (small due to his height and build and giant because of his professional stature), the Japanese surgeon is known for his pioneering work in biliary atresia. The treatment of infants born with the rare disorder, biliary atresia, designed by him won him acclaim all over the world and the surgery known as the Kasai procedure bears his name.

Kasai was born in 1922, in Aomori Prefecture in Japan. He studied medicine in Sendai at the National Tohoku University School of Medicine during tough times, just as the Second World War had ended. After graduating in 1947, he stayed on at the university for his surgical training. Later he joined the 2nd department of surgery at the institution and began working as a general surgeon. At this time, paediatric surgery was not a separate specialty in Japan. However, since Kasai was really interested in paediatrics, he worked on a number of cases where small children required surgery.

Biliary atresia was considered a life-threatening disease for neonates. In the 1950s, the Japanese surgeon was engrossed in comprehending the pathologic processes of the rare disease, leading to cholestasis and eventually cirrhosis. After understanding the disorder in-depth, he devised a surgical intervention plan. The hepatic portoenterostomy technique has been widely credited to him and is popularly known as the Kasai procedure. According to the *Journal of Pediatric Surgery*, 'In 1955, he performed the first Kasai procedure in a 72-day-old infant, who was diagnosed with biliary atresia. During the procedure, Dr Kasai noted no evidence of extrahepatic bile ducts and after further dissection encountered significant bleeding. In an attempt to achieve hemostasis, he is purported to have placed the duodenum over the porta hepatis in the incised region where the bleeding appeared to originate. All were astonished at the appearance of bile pigment in the faeces postoperatively and with the eventual complete resolution of jaundice.' Four years later the procedure found its first mention in the Japanese journal *Shujutsu*.

Eager to hone his skills in paediatric surgery, he completed a 1-year research fellowship in 1959 with Charles Everett Koop, the surgeon-in-chief at the Children's Hospital of Philadelphia. After the fellowship, he dedicated himself full-time and wholeheartedly to the surgery of children. He would return to Koop in Philadelphia to demonstrate the Kasai Procedure at the hospital, which then gained acceptance and popularity in the Western world. After returning to Japan, Kasai was promoted to associate professor of surgery at Tohoku University. Later in 1963 he was promoted to full professor and chief of the 2nd department of surgery, continuing at the university till he retired at the age of 63. Not one to stay home idle, he joined the NTT Tohoku Hospital in 1986, serving as its director till 1993.

Unfortunately, he suffered a stroke in 1999 and the long process of rehabilitation began, lasting nine years. Eventually he passed away in 2008, at the age of 86.

[8]
TEHEMTON UDWADIA

Regarded by many as the 'Father of laparascopic surgery in India', Tehemton Udwadia was the first to perform a surgery using this technique in 1972. In 1990, he also became the first surgeon to perform laparoscopic gall bladder removal in the developing world. With over six decades of experience in medicine, he spent a major part of his career Breach Candy Hospital and Hinduja Hospital, both in Mumbai. He has served as the founder president of the Indian Association of Gastrointestinal Endosurgeons. Udwadia has also been associated with the International College of Surgeons as president of its Indian chapter and world body. An educator par excellence, he takes great pride in knowing that his students and residents are performing challenging surgeries.

Born into a Parsi family in 1934 in Bombay, Udwadia always found early inspiration in his father who was a general practitioner. He completed his early education in Mumbai at St. Mary's School and Wilson College. He graduated in medicine from Mumbai University in 1956 and began working as a research fellow at the King Edward Memorial Hospital. In 1958 he switched to Seth Gordhandas Sunderdas Medical College and stayed on till 1962 whilst also completing his postgraduate degree (MS), for which he qualified in 1960. In 1963 he joined Sir Jamshedjee Jeejeebhoy Group of Hospitals as an assistant professor of surgery. The association was a long one as he was eventually honoured with the emeritus professor status. This would also later become the site where the developing world's first laparoscopy cholecystectomy was performed in 1990. Another feather in his cap was serving as a Hunterian Professor of the Royal College of Surgeons of England in 1984. In 1992, he was the Sir James Ross Lecturer at the Royal College of Surgeons of Edinburgh in 1992.

Udwadia has authored two books on the laparascopy techniques, titled *Laparoscopic Cholecystectomy* and *Laparoscopic Surgery in Developing Countries*. Having been associated with editorial boards of several international journals, he has served as the editor of the *Indian Journal of Surgery* and editor-in-chief of *Journal of Minimal Access Surgery*. In 2000, the Medical Council of India awarded him with the Dr B.C. Roy Award while the Society of American Gastrointestinal Endoscopic Surgeons presented him with the SAGES Millennium Award. In 2006, he was honoured with the Padma Shri, the fourth highest civilian honour in India. In 2017 the Padma Bhushan, which is the third highest civilian honour, was presented to him.

Udwadia is currently associated with Breach Candy Hospital and Hinduja Hospital in Mumbai.

[9]
THEODOR BILLROTH

Widely considered the founder of modern abdominal surgery, Theodor Billroth dabbled with various specialties. However, in his days hardly any specialties were structured and established so he had a free hand. To his credit are a number of firsts in surgery. He was first to remove a portion of the esophagus in 1872 and performed the first complete excision of a larynx in 1873. Billroth pioneered the study of the bacterial causes of wound fever and knew that using antiseptic techniques in surgeries was the answer. He was a fearless, daring and inquisitive surgeon who would alter the size of organs or remove them completely. These were mostly organs that were deemed inaccessible before his escapades.

Born in 1829, in Bergen auf Rügen in the Kingdom of Prussia, Billroth completed his school education in Greifswald. In 1848, he began studying medicine at the University of Greifswald, though he never finished as he gave up in the first term to study music. He finally pursued medicine at the University of Göttingen, and finally earned his medical doctorate in 1852 at the University of Berlin. For the seven years he served as an assistant in B.R.K. Langenbeck's surgical clinic in Berlin. His next appointment took him to Zurich in Switzerland in 1860 where he worked as professor of surgery and director of the surgical clinic at the University of Zurich. In 1867, he moved to Vienna where he was appointed as professor of surgery, and thus began the most exciting phase of his career.

He mastered intestinal surgery in the coming years and in 1881 embarked on the challenging excision of a cancerous pylorus on the lower part of the stomach. He emerged successful and kick-started the modern era of surgery. According to the *Journal of the Balkan Union of Oncology*, 'In Vienna he created one of the finest schools in the history of surgery where he carried out pioneering work in experimental studies, surgical pathology and operative surgery. He pioneered gastric surgery for cancer. In 1881 he carried out the first successful partial gastrectomy for cancer. The first pylorectomy was carried out in 1879 by Jules Péan of Paris but his patient died on the fifth postoperative day.'

For his surgical prowess Billroth was honoured with several awards and titles. However, the rarest honour was the most admirable – in 1887 he was named a member of the Austrian House of Lords, a feat achieved by only a few in his profession.

He died in 1894 at the age of 64.

[10]
LUBOMYR KUZMAK

Inventor of the adjustable silicon band, Lubomyr Kuzmak's innovation revolutionized bariatric surgery.

His invention was approved for as many as seven patents in the USA and seven internationally. The Ukranian surgeon was an active member of the American Society for Bariatric Surgery since its inception in the early 1980s when it was established by the pioneer of obesity surgery Edward Mason. A revered name in the community, he worked hard to promote the budding specialty.

Born in 1929, in Baligrod, Poland, Kuzmak was an excellent student with a keen interest in sports. In 1953 he graduated from the medical school in Lodz, Poland. The site of his postgraduate studies in surgery was the Bytom campus of the Silesian University. After joining the faculty of the university in 1961 he earned himself a degree of Doctor of Science in 1965. By this time, Kuzmak had made up his mind and decided to move to USA. For the next few years he was engaged as a resident and chief resident in general surgery at Saint Barnabas Medical Center in Livingston in New Jersey. In 1971, he began private practice in the same area, finally establishing the Surgical Center for Obesity at Irvington General Hospital in 1981.

In 1983, he invented an adjustable silicon band reinforced with Dacron. It also had a buckle to adjust according to requirement. To install the band in the stomach for obesity surgery, he also equipped the package with a banding instrument and calibrating tube with electronic sensors. He applied for a US patent for the inflatable device, which was approved in 1986. According to the journal *Obesity Surgery*, 'He positioned the band between the short gastric vessels (creating a pouch larger than is accepted nowadays), and also sutured the stomach over the band to prevent slippage. In 1986, he published results in two journals.' He also presented studies spanning seven years covering results of his surgery. He travelled the world to promote his invention and also trained numerous surgeons in the proper use of the adjustable band.

The band was later modified in order to be implanted through the use of laparascopic technology. It popularly came to be known as the lap band while the surgery came to be known as lap band surgery.

He died in 2006, succumbing to pneumonia.

FIVE

HIGHEST RATED TRANSPLANT SURGEONS

MANKIND HAS ALWAYS BEEN FASCINATED WITH replacing that which is not functional. The history of organ transplantation is no different and dates back to 1869 when the first skin transplant was performed. Through years of trial and error, the medical fraternity has come to a relatively comfortable phase when organ transplants, though not a cakewalk, are certainly safer and more feasible than they were 50 years ago. The development of sophisticated anti-rejection drugs, a result of labourous hours in the labs by researchers, have played a major role in making organ transplants a viable option and far less intimidating than they used to be. Today we know a lot more about the immune system and its responses, and possess the ability to manipulate it to our advantage.

However, a major challenge that no technological advancement has been able to achieve is the lack of donors. There is a major discrepancy between the number of donors and needy recipients. And as of now, artificially created organs in the lab still have a long way to go. On the bright side, exciting events are happening in the transplant specialty and it's not just the organs but innovations in hand, leg and even face replacements are also coming to the fore. Surgeons and researchers are working hand in hand with technology to achieve what was once unfathomable.

[1]
JEAN-MICHEL DUBERNARD

Liver and pancreas transplants are passé for this innovative transplant surgeon. Transplants that add mobility and functionality to a patient by replacing hands and feet, limbs and even the face are what excites Jean-Michel Dubernard. In 1998, he became the first surgeon to conduct the transplant of a single human hand successfully. Shortly after his first success, he conducted a double hand transplant the same year, however, the results were only made public in 2004. The wait was probably to analyse the long-term effects and efficacy of the transplant. In 2005 he undertook the challenge of assisting French maxillofacial surgeon Bernard Devauchelle in the first partial face transplant. The recipient's face was destroyed when she was mauled by a dog.

Born in 1941 in Lyon, France, Dubernard completed his medical studies at Lyon Medical School in 1965. He then flew to USA to study at Harvard Medical School in Boston, passing out in 1967, simultaneously achieving his Doctor of Medicine at the University of Lyon. He also became Doctor of Philosophy from the University of Lyon in 1971. In 1976, he performed the first pancreas transplant in France. Since 1977 he has been the professor of urological surgery at the University of Lyon. From 1979 to 2007, he was appointed as the chief of the department of urology and transplant surgery at the Edouard Herriot Hospital, Lyon. Since 2008, he was placed in the position of chairman at the medium devices assessment committee.

For the hush-hush double hand transplant in 1998, the French surgeon had organised a 16-hour procedure aided by a team of 16 surgeons and 20 nurses. A psychoanalyst was also part of the transplant team to counsel the patient on the psychological considerations of having an external, visible body part operated on. According to the results published in the *Annals of Surgery* in 2003, 'The recipient was a 33-year-old man with bilateral amputation. Surgery included procurement of the upper extremities from a multiorgan cadaveric donor, preparation of the graft and recipient's stumps; then, bone fixation, arterial and venous anastomoses, nerve sutures, joining of tendons and muscles and skin closure. Rehabilitation programme included physiotherapy, electrostimulation and occupational therapy. Immunosuppressive protocol included tacrolimus, prednisone and mycophenolate mofetil and, for induction, antithymocyte globulins and then CD25 monoclonal antibody were added. Sensorimotor recovery tests and functional magnetic resonance imaging (fMRI) were performed to assess functional return and cortical reorganization. All the results were classified according to Ipsen's classification.'

The French surgeon's life also led him to dabble in politics. A member of the French National Assembly from 1986 to 2007, Dubernard keeps himself busy with continuous transplant research work. He has been decorated with honours such as the Ordre National du Mérite, Ordre des Palmes Académiques.

[2]
SIR ROY YORKE CALNE

One of the most formidable names in organ transplant surgery, Sir Roy Yorke Calne pursued the specialty when the popular opinion was not much in its favour. He took up the challenge of conducting organ transplants in the mid-1950s for patients suffering from end-stage organ failure who could no longer be helped with medication and lifestyle changes. The chances of the surgery working were low, but such patients were willing to take the risk. One of the most valuable contributions of the British surgeon was establishing an internationally renowned kidney and liver transplant programme at Addenbrooke's Hospital in Cambridge in 1965. Calne took up the initiative when he was appointed professor of surgery at the University of Cambridge.

Born in 1930 in Surrey, Calne graduated from Lancing College in West Sussex and obtained his medical training at King's College's GKT Medical School of Education and Guy's Hospital Medical School, both in London. He was also involved in the National Service, travelling to Hong Kong, Singapore and Malaysia for the same.

He worked with various hospitals in London and also held surgical appointments at Harvard Medical School. In 1965, he was appointed professor of surgery in the University of Cambridge. Calne was elected fellow of the Royal Society in 1974.

He performed the first liver transplant procedure in Europe in 1968. In 1987, the world stood up in awe at the procedure he conducted – the world's first simultaneous multiorgan transplant. In collaboration with a cardiothoracic surgeon, Calne undertook a liver, heart and lung transplant. He was also the first to perform an intestinal transplant in the UK in 1992. In 1994 he outdid himself by performing the first successful combined stomach, intestine, pancreas, liver and kidney cluster transplant.

The pioneering surgeon, in one of his papers published in the journal *Science Progress*, discussed the scenario, talking about the challenges he faced. 'Organ transplantation started in the mid-1950s with a kidney transplant between identical twins, demonstrating the surgical technique could provide successful therapy. The immunological barrier to be overcome, however, proved to be far more difficult to deal with. The introduction of immunosuppressive agents produced some success but it was not until Cyclosporin became available in the 1980s that results became sufficiently good for widespread acceptance and rapid development of organ grafting. Now with more powerful and selective agents, although there is still much room for improvement in immunosuppression, one of the main problems in organ transplantation is a result of its success, namely a shortage of organ donors.'

Calne has earned various awards and honours. He was knighted by the Queen in 1986. Other noteworthy awards include the Cameron Prize for Therapeutics of the University of Edinburgh, Ernst Jung Prize, Prince Mahidol Award and Pride of Britain Lifetime Achievement Award. In 2012, he shared the esteemed Lasker Award (Lasker-DeBakey Clinical Medical Research Award) with Thomas Starzl 'for the development of liver transplantation, which has restored normal life to thousands of patients with end-stage liver disease.'

At the age of 90 he is retired but remains abreast of the times with all that's new in his specialty.

[3]
PEDRO CAVADAS

The pioneering Spanish surgeon redefined transplant surgery by introducing the world to the novel concept of intervention surgery. Such an approach to surgery incorporates all means necessary to keep a limb or organ functional or use transplantation techniques in such a way that it benefits the patient without being typically identical to their current anatomy. This approach has earned Pedro Cavadas a reputation as one of the most distinctive and innovative surgeons. Though technically a plastic and reconstructive surgeon, he is well-revered in limb transplants and is an authority on microsurgery. His groundbreaking approach converted a patient's right hand into his left hand. The right side of the patient's body had become disabled. By transplanting these hands, now technically located in a new position, the surgeon allowed the patient to still use his good hand. Cavadas has also undertaken surgeries to transplant a patient's arm onto their leg to keep it alive during a procedure. The radical strategy saved the arm for later use.

Born in Valencia in 1965, Cavadas completed most of his medical education at the University of Valencia, earning his medical degree in 1989 and PhD in 1995. After medical school, he completed his residency in the La Fe Hospital in Valencia, becoming a specialist in plastic and reconstructive surgery. He has been heading the Hospital of Manises Dr Cavadas Microsurgical and Reconstructive Surgery Unit since 2011. Working closely with a team of three surgeons under him, he performs roughly 1,800 surgeries every year. He specialises in unusual cases wherein patients have been rejected from surgery or have disabilities that are extremely complicated to repair.

Among the many surgical feats achieved by Cavadas is the case of Alba Lucía Carmona as he sewed back on both her hands. Interestingly, about 70 per cent of hand transplants have chances of being unsuccessful as they may face rejection and infection. However, Carmona recovered significantly well regaining a great degree of mobility in her hands. In 2018, he also achieved similar success with a US Naval officer. Cavadas has also developed the perforator flaps SS-PTP, M-SAP, BiFeP and more.

In 2003, the Pedro Cavadas Foundation was launched by him. It provides modern reconstructive surgery solutions to underprivileged patients in Africa. He has won awards such as the International Ibero-Latin-American Federation prize for Residents in Plastic Surgery and the senior resident prize for Plastic Surgery Residents in Microsurgery of the American Society of Plastic Surgeons in the USA.

[4]
JOSEPH MURRAY

The pioneering plastic surgeon is considered the father of organ transplantation in USA. In 1990, Joseph Murray received the coveted Nobel Prize for Physiology or Medicine (with co-winner E. Donnall Thomas) for his commendable work in tissue and organ transplantation techniques. The prize was the culmination of years of hard work, labour and research. Murray's tenacious spirit didn't not allow him to quit and he continued his experiments for more than a decade before tasting success in 1954 when he conducted the world's first successful human kidney transplant on identical twins Richard and Ronald Herrick.

Murray was born in 1919 in Milford, Massachusetts, USA. He obtained a bachelor of arts degree from Holy Cross College, Worcester, Massachusetts, in 1940, followed by a medical degree from Harvard Medical School, Cambridge, Massachusetts, in 1943. He was a surgical resident thereafter at Peter Bent Brigham Hospital in Boston, where his prize-winning research would begin.

During the Second World War, when he was inducted into the medical corps of the US Army, he made an observation that would consume his thoughts. While working in the plastic surgery unit in Pennsylvania, he observed that skin grafts were successful only between identical twins. The burn victims' bodies would mostly reject skin grafts from unrelated donors. He wondered if the rationale would also work for transplanted internal organs and he started experimenting with kidney transplants in dogs.

After the war he resumed working at the Peter Bent Brigham Hospital and in 1954 he performed a kidney transplant. The patient's identical twin had offered to donate a kidney and Murray finally had a chance to support his theory. The operation was a resounding success. The donor as well as the recipient survived for several decades after the procedure. However, not everyone who needs a transplant has an identical or even fraternal twin. He kept at his research, looking for ways to suppress the immune system so that it wouldn't reject genetically foreign parts. Using immunosuppressive drugs, in 1962 he conducted the first successful kidney transplant wherein the donor was unrelated to the patient. Later, he would manage to harvest a kidney from a cadaver and transplant it into a patient.

Starting from 1964 Murray worked as chief plastic surgeon at Peter Bent Brigham. In 1972 he was also appointed chief plastic surgeon at Children's Hospital Boston. He continued in both these roles for over a decade. In 1970 he became professor of surgery at Harvard Medical School, retiring in 1986 as professor emeritus.

Murray published an autobiography in 2001 called *Surgery of the Soul: Reflections on a Curious Career*. It was widely acclaimed in the medical community.

Apart from the Nobel Prize, Murray also received the American Surgical Association's Medal for Distinguished Service to Surgery, the American Academy of Arts and Sciences' Francis Amory Prize, the American Association of Plastic Surgeons' Honorary Award and Clinician of the Year Award, the National Kidney Foundation's Gift of Life Award and the Golden Plate Award of the American Academy of Achievement, among other honours.

He passed away in 2012 at Peter Bent Brigham Hospital where it had all started, after suffering a brief illness.

[5]
LALL SAWH

The urologist surgeon who brought organ transplant to Trinidad and Tobago was the first to conduct a kidney transplant procedure in the Caribbean. The donor and recipient were living and related. Among Lall Sawh's other firsts are being one of the first surgeons in the region to perform minimally invasive surgeries, introducing the 'buttonhole' kidney surgery, and using the Dornier lithotripter, a machine that pulverises kidney stones by means of shock waves.

Born in the town of Couva in Trinidad and Tobago, Sawh was motivated to become a doctor after seeing the demise of his brother who bled to death as his jugular vein had been cut. With monetary help from his pharmacist uncle, he began his medical studies in 1968 at the age of 17 at the University of the West Indies, Jamaica where he graduated with first class honours. He went on to receive the Commonwealth Scholarship from the United Kingdom. The training programme had him go through rotations at the Royal Infirmary of Edinburgh in Scotland and then at the Institute of Urology in London, England.

After specializing in urology in the UK, he was back in his country which, after gaining independence in 1962, had become a republic in the commonwealth of nations in 1976. Several doctors left the country, including two urologists, leaving him as the only urologist left in the country. It was now upon him to develop the budding specialty. He pioneered numerous urological procedures at the San Fernando General Hospital in Trinidad.

In 1985, he trained in USA and began training as a Laparoscopic and Endoscopic Urology fellow at the Mayo Clinic in Rochester, Minnesota. He would soon introduce what he learnt at the Mayo Clinic in the Caribbean. This was followed by further training at the Urology Department at Washington University in St. Louis, Missouri. In 1988 he conducted the first set of kidney transplants in Trinidad and Tobago. He further honed his skills with more transplant trainings in the US. He went on to work on several high profile cases including several political heads and even presidents and prime ministers.

Sawh has been featured in lists like 'Who's Who in the World of Science and Technology' and '100 Greatest Living Surgeons'. At 43 he was the youngest winner of the Chaconia Gold Medal, Trinidad and Tobago's highest honour for excellence in medicine and surgery. The government of the country has awarded him with the national award and named him a national icon. He was also honoured by the Society of Surgeons in Trinidad and Tobago. His name was featured as one of the few surgeons, in Nasser Khan's historical recount, 'Profiles – Heroes, Pioneers and Role Models of Trinidad and Tobago' in 2012. He was also enlisted as one of the 12 people who helped transform Trinidad and Tobago in 2018.

He is currently involved in private practices at Southern Medical Clinic in south Trinidad and at West Shore Medical in west Trinidad. He also serves as an associate lecturer at the University of the West Indies.

[6] MEHMET HABERAL

An iconic figure in the medical community in Turkey, Mehmet Haberal is not only a pioneer in transplant surgery in his country, but is also the founder of Başkent University in Ankara. He trained under the legendary American organ transplant surgeon Thomas Starzl, assisting him in cases of several of the longest surviving early liver transplant patients. Haberal was a key player and worked extensively on the legislation concerning the harvesting, storage, grafting and transplantation of organs and tissues that was passed by the Turkish parliament in 1979. This act lent structure and stability to the practice of transplantation procedures in the country.

Haberal was born in Pazar, a small town along the Black Sea in Turkey. In 1967 he graduated from Ankara University Medical School located in Ankara, Turkey. The same year he became a resident in the department of surgery at Hacettepe University Faculty of Medicine, rising to the rank of general surgeon specialist in 1971. He was off to the US to complete a fellowship at Shriner's Burns Institute and the John Sealy Hospital in

Galveston, Texas, in 1973. The next year he completed another fellowship in the USA at the Colorado University Medical School Transplantation Center. Upon returning to Turkey, he set up the burn and transplantation unit in 1975 at Hacettepe University Hospital, department of general surgery.

Hereon, Haberal's career was dotted with firsts. In 1975 he conducted the first living-related kidney transplant in Turkey. The kidney was donated from a mother to her son aged 12. In 1978, he became the first person to perform a kidney transplant harvested from a cadaver in Turkey. He was the first to conduct a successful cadaver liver transplantation in 1988 in Turkey, the Middle East and Northern Africa. In 1992, he set another record by becoming the first to conduct the first combined liver–kidney transplantation from a living-related donor in the world.

He was the man behind the creation of several professional societies like the Middle East Society for Organ Transplantation (MESOT); Middle East Dialysis and Organ Transplantation Foundation (MEDOTF); and Turkish Transplantation Society. In 1993 he established the Başkent University in Ankara. With over 2000 publications to his credit, he has also authored six book and earned several honorary fellowships and doctorates from around the world.

Some of the most prestigious awards presented to him have been the Everett Idris Evans Memorial Award from the American Burn Association in 1985; Distinguished Philanthropist Award by the American College of Surgeons in 2017 and Lifetime Achievement Award by Kuwaiti Minister of Health, Shaikh Ahmad Al-Abdulla Al-Sabah in 2006.

He is currently engaged in politics and is a member of the Turkish Parliament.

[7]
SIR MICHAEL WOODRUFF

Known for pioneering organ transplant in the United Kingdom, Sir Michael Woodruff also conducted ground breaking research in the field. An academic surgeon, he was consumed by research in the subject of transplant rejection and immunosuppression, and even invented a drug to prevent rejection in such procedures. His research culminated in the first kidney transplant on identical twins in 1960 in the United Kingdom at Edinburgh's Royal Infirmary. Though the procedure came with its own set of complications, it was ultimately successful with both the donor and recipient surviving.

Born in Mill Hill in London in 1911, Woodruff grew up in Australia and attended the Trinity Grammar School in Melbourne. Winning a government scholarship to the University of Melbourne and Queen's College, Woodruff decided to study electrical engineering and mathematics, graduating in 1933. He later went to medical school at the

University of Melbourne and graduated in 1938. For one year after graduation he studied internal medicine, serving as house surgeon at the Royal Melbourne Hospital. He completed his Master of Surgery in Melbourne and also joined the Royal Australian Medical Corps during the Second World War, when he was captured by the Japanese along with many others.

After coming to Britain in 1946, he took up a teaching position in surgery at Sheffield University and was elected a fellow of the Royal College of Surgeons of England. He spent the next part of his career working in Aberdeen, and then in 1952, he moved to Dunedin, New Zealand where he was appointed professor of surgery at the University of Otago. In 1957, Woodruff was back in the UK joining the University of Edinburgh as professor of surgery and the Royal Infirmary. All this while he was conducting research on organ transplantation but was quite wary of the phenomena of rejection.

It was at the Royal Infirmary where the UK's first ever kidney transplant took place. Woodruff's wait for the ideal patient who had an identical twin to act as the donor had ended. With such a donor–recipient profile, the risk of rejection would be minimized to a great extent. The patient, a 49-year-old man with acutely impaired kidney function was operated upon and transplanted with his twin brother's kidney. The brothers lived for six years after the disease and died due to an unrelated condition.

He wrote several papers and eight books, of which

one was on transplantation and was held in high esteem for many years. Elected a fellow of the Royal Society in 1968, Woodruff was knighted by the Queen the next year in 1969. He enjoyed the honorary memberships of the American College of Surgeons, the American Surgical Association, the Royal College of Physicians of Edinburgh and more. He also served as an advisor to the World Health Organization for a few years.

He died in 2001 at the age of 89.

[8]
ARVINDER SINGH SOIN

A pioneer of liver transplant in India, Arvinder Singh Soin has conducted more than 2,500 liver transplants – a record of sorts. He also has several national and global firsts to his credit, such as first successful cadaveric liver transplant in India in 1998; first successful long distance cadaveric liver transplant wherein the liver was transported by air from Chennai to be transplanted in New Delhi in 1999; and the first successful combined liver and kidney transplant in India in 1999, among others. In 2005, he performed the first bloodless liver transplant. In the same year Soin also undertook the first successful emergency liver transplant on a patient who was in a deep coma and was transferred to New Delhi by air ambulance. Using organs from two different donors, he conducted liver and kidney transplants on the same patient in 2007. This surgery was the first of its kind in the world.

Soin was born in Birmingham in the United Kingdom in 1963. After completing his MBBS in 1985 and MS in 1989 from All India Institute of Medical Sciences in New Delhi, he was off to the UK. Here in 1993, he completed a fellowship at the Royal College of Surgeons of Edinburgh followed by another one at the Royal College of Physicians and Surgeons of Glasgow. He trained in liver and biliary surgery, liver and kidney transplant surgery, small bowel/intestinal transplant and pancreas transplant, staying on in the UK for six years. He also served as surgical tutor and faculty in the University of Cambridge. In 1997 he also went through training in transplant surgery at the Royal College of Surgeons, before making his way back to India. Here he could put his experience to good use and established liver transplantation in the country.

He began working with Apollo Hospital and Sir Gangaram Hospital. In 2001 he worked tirelessly to set up a state-of-the-art liver transplant centre at Sir Gangaram Hospital – a process that almost took a decade. In 2010, he joined Medanta – The Medicity, in Gurugram. Soin is a part of several pertinent societies such as the National Advisory Board in Liver Transplantation, British Transplantation Society, Indian Society of Organ Transplantation, Indian Society of Gastroenterology Indian Association of Surgical Gastroenterology, Indian

Society of Nephrology, Asian Living Donor Liver Transplant Group and Asia Pacific Organ Transplant Forum. Soin has also earned several honours like the Delhi Medical Association Distinguished Service Awards in 2005 and 2010, Padma Shri by the President of India in 2010 and the RD Birla 2011 Outstanding Clinician of the year.

He serves as the Chief Hepatobiliary and Liver Transplant Surgeon and Chairman, Medanta Institute of Liver Transplantation and Regenerative Medicine at Medanta – The Medcity in Gurugram, Delhi NCR.

[9]
SIR TERENCE ENGLISH

He was a daring surgeon who turned things around for transplant surgery in the United Kingdom. Heart transplant surgery had trickled into the country after South African surgeon Christiaan Barnard had performed it for the first time in 1967. Everyone wanted to try it. However, with poor survival rates, a moratorium had been placed on heart transplantation in the country. The funding would be cut off and Sir Terence English had the last chance to keep heart transplantation surgeries alive in the UK. In 1979 he performed Britain's first successful heart transplant, changing the course for the specialty in the country.

Born in 1932 in Pietermaritzburg in South Africa,

English always had a scientific bend of mind and pursued a degree in Mining Engineering in Johannesburg's Witwatersrand University. He then switched to medicine, partly inspired by his uncle who was a surgeon. He was accepted at Guy's Hospital Medical School in London. He passed out in 1962 and began his surgical training, first in general surgery and then in cardiothoracic surgery at the Royal Brompton Hospital, and London Chest and National Heart Hospitals.

In 1972, English joined Papworth and Addenbrooke's Hospitals of the University of Cambridge as consultant cardiothoracic surgeon. Heart transplantation became his major surgical interest and he would apply all he had learned under leading surgeons like Donald Ross and Sir Russell, later Lord Brock, under whom he had trained. He had also visited Christiaan Barnard in South Africa. In 1979, he performed the first successful heart transplant in the country and the recipient lived a good life for over five years. There was no looking back after that. English worked with the Papworth and Addenbrooke's hospitals till 1995. He was appointed director of the British Heart Foundation Research Group at Papworth in 1980. The hospital became an international hub for heart, heart–lung and lung transplantation under his able leadership. In 1986, English would go on to conduct the UK's first total artificial heart transplant – a stop gap arrangement till a suitable human donor was found.

English was a part of several prestigious professional

societies and served as the president of the Royal College of Surgeons of England from 1989 to 1992, and president of the British Medical Association in 1995. He became Master of St. Catharine's College in Cambridge in 1993 till 2000. He earned several awards and accolades for his distinguished service, and was made Knight Commander of the British Empire in 1991. Other notable awards presented to him include the Clement Price Thomas Award by the Royal College of Surgeons of England; Lifetime Achievement Award by the Society for Cardiothoracic Surgery in Great Britain and Ireland; Lifetime Achievement Award from the International Society for Heart and Lung Transplantation in recognition of outstanding achievements and tireless dedication in the field of heart and lung transplantation.

Now retired, English lives with his wife in Oxford.

[10]
MOHAMED RELA

This Indian surgeon gathered praise and acclaim when he successfully transplanted the liver of a baby who was merely five days old in the year 2000. The baby is now in her twenties and pursuing law in Ireland. He has established an expertise in liver transplants involving small children with complicated liver issues with no other solution except a transplant. After spending a significant portion of his career in the UK, he returned to India and has now set up his own medical centre and institute in Chennai. He has researched extensively on the role of nitric oxide in chronic allograft rejection, ischemia reperfusion, liver gene therapy and biliary atresia.

Born in 1959 in the small village of Kiliyanur near Mayiladuthurai in Tamil Nadu, India, Rela completed his MBBS in 1982 and MS in 1987 from the University of Madras. In 1988 he completed a fellowship at the Royal College of Surgeons of Edinburgh, United Kingdom. In 2013, he received an honorary degree from the Tamil Nadu Dr MGR Medical University in India.

Rela trained in several hospitals in the UK. Finally, in 1991 he joined King's College Hospital in London. He pioneered several specialized liver transplantation techniques at King's College Hospital such as auxiliary transplantation and live donor liver transplantation. In the late 2000s, he returned to India, working in a number of hospitals in Chennai. He set up the Institute of Liver Disease and Transplantation at Global Gleneagles Health City in 2009. In 2018 he started his own venture, Dr Rela Institute and Medical Centre in Chennai.

Rela has won several awards and is a member of the British Medical Association, Royal Society of Medicine, British Transplantation Society, International Liver Transplant Society, Association of Upper GI Surgeons of Great Britain, European Society of Organ

Transplantation and British Association of Study of the Liver. He was also the president-elect 2021 for the International Liver Transplant Society.

Rela currently serves as the chairman and director at the Dr Rela Institute and Medical Centre, Chennai. He also serves as the professor of liver surgery and transplantation at the Institute of Liver Disease King's College Hospital, London.